THE KNEE
Clinical Applications

A.L. LOGAN SERIES IN CHIROPRACTIC TECHNIQUE

The Knee: Clinical Applications
The Foot and Ankle: Clinical Applications
The Low Back and Pelvis: Clinical Applications

THE KNEE
Clinical Applications

A.L. Logan
Series in
Chiropractic
Technique

Alfred L. Logan

With a contribution by
Lindsay J. Rowe

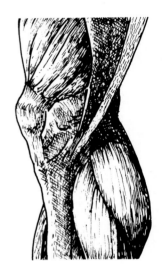

Alfred L. Logan, DC
Formerly associated with
Los Angeles College of Chiropractic
Whittier, California
and
Anglo-European College Of Chiropractic
Bournemouth, England

**Lindsay J. Rowe, MAppSc (Chiropractic),
MD, DACBR (USA), FCCR (CAN),
FACCR (AUST), FICC**
Newcastle, Australia

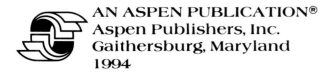
AN ASPEN PUBLICATION®
Aspen Publishers, Inc.
Gaithersburg, Maryland
1994

Library of Congress Cataloging-in-Publication Data
Logan, Alfred L.
The knee: clinical applications/Alfred L. Logan.
p. cm. — (A.L. Logan series in chiropractic technique)
Includes bibliographical references and index.
ISBN: 0-8342-0522-X
1. Knee—Diseases—Chiropractic treatment.
2. Knee—Wounds and injuries—Chiropractic treatment.
I. Title. II. Series.
[DNLM: 1. Knee Injuries—diagnosis. 2. Knee Injuries—therapy.
3. Knee—physiopathology. 4. Chiropractic—methods. WE 870
L831k 1994]
RZ265.K53L64 1994
617.5'82—dc20
DNLM/DLC
for Library of Congress
93-39114
CIP

The author has made every effort to ensure the accuracy of the information
herein. However, appropriate information sources should be consulted, especially for new or unfamiliar procedures. It is the responsibility of every practitioner to evaluate the appropriateness of a particular opinion in the context of
actual clinical situations and with due consideration to new developments. The
author, editors, and the publisher cannot be held responsible for any typographi-
cal or other errors found in this book.

Editorial Resources: Amy Martin

Library of Congress Catalog Card Number: 93-39114
ISBN: 0-8342-0522-X

Printed in the United States of America

1 2 3 4 5

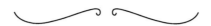

Anyone who has been to school can remember at least one teacher whose influence inspired him to learn more fully, to appreciate the subject being taught, and perhaps to realize a life's work. I have been fortunate enough to have had several such teachers. In high school, my biology teacher moved me into the sciences, and a humanities teacher instilled in me the desire to think and reason. While studying chiropractic, I found Dr. A.L. Logan. I first met him when he voluntarily did clinical rounds at the Los Angeles College of Chiropractic.

Roy Logan had a capacity to understand how the human body works, and a curiosity about it that kept him constantly searching and researching for ways to help heal it. The profession is full of personalities teaching a variety of techniques, some insisting theirs is the only way, but it has few true professors who can cull the various teachings, and present to the student a clear and concise way to approach a patient, without personality and ego getting in the way. Roy had these abilities, and, fortunately for us, he had a desire to teach others. He never missed an opportunity.

He saw the need in our profession for a way to link the rote clinical sciences and the various ways of executing an adjustment. He gave us an answer to the commonly asked question of when and where to adjust. He was constantly pushing the profession to realize the importance of effective clinical application of chiropractic principles at a time when there seemed to be more emphasis on fitting into the health care industry by wearing a white coat and using big words.

Around the world, students of Dr. Logan use his methods of diagnosis and treatment every day and are reminded of his wonderful contributions to the profession. He lectured repeatedly before several state associations, and taught an eight month post-graduate course at LACC for eight years. He was Chairman of the Technique Department at the Anglo-European College of Chiropractic for five years.

In spite of his many contributions, Roy's work remains unfinished. He passed away in April of 1993, after fighting a terminal illness. He was working hard on his textbooks up to the end, hoping to transfer as much of his knowledge and wisdom to paper as he could.

Dr. Logan has a number of students dedicated to continuing his work and seeing it evolve in the way he envisioned. There is no "A.L. Logan Technique," but rather a compilation of various teachings, combined with a unique understanding of the interdependencies of the human structure. We hope to do his work justice and see more students of chiropractic become as effective as possible in the treatment of human disorders.

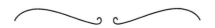

Table of Contents

Foreword

Helping patients, teaching students and practitioners how to assess and evaluate the problems of patients, and arriving at optimal treatment plans were some of the late Dr. Roy Logan's goals. This book provides the reader with a systematic approach to carrying out an assessment and understanding the reasons behind the various aspects of treatment.

The Knee: Clinical Applications follows an orderly progression from the anatomy of the knee through examination, including muscle testing, with many illustrations and a chapter on imaging. Adjustive techniques are also illustrated completely, as are the chapters addressing conditions of the knee, therapy, and exercise.

The chapter on case histories draws on some of Dr. Logan's most interesting clinical experiences; they demonstrate the art of problem solving. The examination chapter is organized in a manner consistent with helping the examiner pinpoint a problem. To complete an assessment the patient must be properly and thoroughly examined. Accurate diagnosis depends on a knowledge of functional anatomy and history, as well as diligent observation. Both background and process are provided here.

Dr. Logan dedicated his professional life to an extensive study of neuromusculoskeletal structure and the biomechanics of the body. This book provides the reader with a thorough understanding of the practical biomechanics of the knee.

I deeply appreciate my friendship with the late Dr. Logan and the opportunity to have spent many delightful hours with him discussing anatomy, biomechanics, and patient assessment, then arriving at an adjustive or manipulative technique supported by our findings and observations. It is my expectation that this text, intended for both students and practitioners, will offer them the same opportunity to increase their professional armamentarium and enhance their clinical understanding.

Herbert I. Magee, Jr., DC, FICC
Redwood City, California

Series Preface

"... The application of principles ... involves higher mental processes than their memorizing; every student should be given a thorough drill in clinical analysis in which he should be made to see the relationship which exists between the fundamental facts and their clinical application."

Francis M. Pottenger, MD

The education that a modern chiropractor undergoes includes the clinical sciences and the manipulative arts. A graduate doctor of chiropractic has a thorough grasp of the diagnostic and clinical skills and is trained in basic manipulative techniques. With this knowledge, the practicing doctor begins to gain the experience that makes the application of this knowledge successful. A successful doctor is one who continues to learn beyond what is minimally required, for he or she is constantly renewed and stimulated.

Dr. A.L. Logan was a successful chiropractor, a doctor that, like D.D. Palmer, continued to expand his understanding of the human body in health and disease. He studied the works of many of the chiropractic profession's leading educators. He researched and developed his own theories which he applied in his practice, and like most chiropractors, developed a successful, diversified approach to diagnosing and treating his patients. Dr. Logan recognized the need for a practical way to blend basic and advanced manipulative techniques with clinical skills.

From this recognition came over 20 years of teaching. It was his hope that his ideas would generate continued dialogue and interest in expanding the clinical application of chiropractic principles.

Dr. Logan did clinical rounds at the Los Angeles College of Chiropractic, since the early seventies. He lectured often for various state associations, and taught at the Anglo-European College of Chiropractic. During this time Dr. Logan continued to learn and grow as a clinician and teacher. His decision to write a series of texts on the clinical application of chiropractic principles came out of his experience in teaching undergraduate technique at AECC and seeing the difficulty upper division students had in understanding when, where, and why they should adjust.

This series of textbooks will be a comprehensive reference on chiropractic clinical applications. Dr. Logan believed this approach should be the basis for an undergraduate course in adjustive and clinical technique. It is, at the same time, a welcome addition to the knowledge of any practitioner.

Pottenger FM. *Symptoms of Visceral Disease*. St. Louis: Mosby; 1953.

Chris Hutcheson, DC
Auburn, California

Preface

The following remarks are the author's. They appear as written
before his untimely death in April 1993.

While I taught postgraduate technique classes at the Los Angeles College of Chiropractic for a number of years, some things became apparent. With students from many chiropractic colleges, the strong points as well as weaknesses of the undergraduate programs were easily noted in workshop. Some programs were totally lacking in extremity techniques. Others placed little emphasis on the extremities, leaving them until the end of the technique program. After teaching postgraduate classes, I had the privilege to teach undergraduate technique for four academic years at the Anglo-European College of Chiropractic in Bournemouth, England. Most of my classes were in the third- and fourth-year program, and most were on the extremities.

All too often the spine and pelvis are taught first and then the extremities. In chiropractic, the emphasis should be on the spine and pelvis and their influence on the body through the nervous system. I have been insisting for many years, however, that teaching the spine and pelvis before the lower extremities makes it extremely difficult for the student to grasp overall functional anatomy.

Being urged to write about my approach to technique, my first consideration was to write about some of the exciting things I have worked with in the last few years (anatomic short leg, lumbosacral techniques, etc). Several of my former students urged me to write what I have been saying for years is the ideal sequence, starting with the knee, moving to the foot, and following with the hip, pelvis, and spine.

Now I have completed this text on what I consider the best place to start: learning to palpate and examine, range of motion, how the muscles feel, how to test them, and how to recognize fixations of the knee. Why? The knee is the largest articulation in the body. It is easy to palpate because it is readily available, and there are two of them. It is easy to learn that both sides may be similar yet may have their unique differences and still be normal. The knee is a less dangerous place to start the beginner than the pelvis or the cervical spine.

I have attempted to write a text suitable for use by the beginner or the practitioner who has never had instruction on the knee. Included are anatomy illustrations emphasizing the clinical viewpoint; these are referred to throughout to help the reader retain the anatomy information while learning how to use it.

Acknowledgments

No book is written without a number of people being involved. The amount of time and effort requires an encroachment on the lives of friends, associates, and family. I would like to thank the following individuals:

My wife, Judy A. Logan, DC, for her many roles over the months; her patience throughout; her encouragement from the beginning to the end; and her hours of reading, commenting on, and editing the text.

Michael Weisenberger, DC, Geelong, Australia, for his encouragement, if not downright insistence, that I write this book, and for his invaluable advice and assistance in this, our first ever computer effort.

Our son, S/Sgt Stephen Hillenbrand, USAF, for his many hours and expertise in producing the photography that made most of the illustrations possible.

A special thanks to Paula Regina Rodriques de Freitas Hillenbrand, our model throughout, for her many hours of posing for us, which made the illustrations possible.

Lindsay J. Rowe, DC, MD, for his invaluable contribution to the text, which allowed coverage of everything except surgery within the one text.

Herbert I. Magee, Jr., DC, for his invaluable assistance in editing the text.

Merrill Cook, DC, for the use of his library, his advice when asked, and his support.

Niels Nilsson, DC, MD, for his suggestions and assistance in editing.

William Remson, DC, for his suggestions and assistance in editing.

Reed B. Phillips, DC, PhD, for reviewing the text and for his suggestions.

Inger F. Villadsen, DC, for her encouragement throughout and for her help in the final edit.

Chris Hutcheson, DC, for his review and editorial support in the later stages of production.

Chapter 1

Anatomy

The ligaments of the normal knee provide stability throughout the full range of motion, allowing even the sometimes spectacular feats seen in sports. The strength of the ligaments and the power of the muscles can be appreciated when we observe a 200-lb person jumping and landing on one limb with the knee bent.

The knee is the largest joint in the body, with most of the structures being relatively easy to locate. For the student, the knee is the ideal joint to begin developing the skills of observation, palpation, and testing.

Not only is the knee large, but it is easily accessible and has sufficient stability to allow safe testing of the range of motion, muscle strength, and orthopedics. The experience of palpating the large, mobile knee should provide the examiner with the basic skills to begin the more complex, difficult examination of the spine and pelvis.

A knowledge of the anatomy is necessary to understand function. The importance of anatomy cannot be stressed too much. In a study the author conducted at the Anglo-European Chiropractic College of students in the second- and third-year program who were having difficulty or failing, it was found that the students had barely managed to pass anatomy in the first year.

Without a thorough understanding of anatomy, reading X-rays, conducting a proper examination, adjusting, and arriving at a proper treatment program are not possible. This chapter on the anatomy will provide the basics of anatomy for the student and a review for the practitioner.

BONY STRUCTURES

The two major bones of the knee are the femur, the longest and strongest bone in the body, and the tibia, the second longest bone. The patella is the largest sesamoid bone in the body (Figure 1–1).

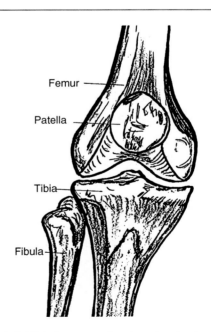

Figure 1–1 Right knee, anterior view showing bony structures.

The distal end of the femur enlarges into two condyles, with articular surfaces allowing articulation inferiorly with the tibia and anteriorly with the patella. The patellar articular surface blends in with and separates into a medial and lateral articular surface, forming a U shape (Figure 1–2).

The lateral femoral condyle is more prominent, projecting anteriorly farther than the medial, and provides a resistance to help prevent the patella from dislocating laterally. Posteriorly the articular surfaces of the femur extend approximately the same distance (Figure 1–3).

The position of the fibula is slightly behind the lateral condyle of the tibia, yet on the surface that angles downward and anteriorly. This prevents direct anterior movement and limits the proximal movement of the fibula.

The medial articular surface of the tibia extends a greater distance anteriorly than laterally, allowing greater movement[1] (Figure 1–4).

Note the extent of the femoral articular surface (Figure 1–5), allowing the normal range of motion of the knee from approximately 5° of hyperextension to 160° of flexion. Some clinicians refer to the –5° to –10° as normal extension. For the purposes of this text, extension is 0° or neutral, and all movement beyond 0° is hyperextension.

The fibula is not a part of the articulation of the knee, but it plays a major role in knee function and must be considered because of the ligament and muscle attachments.

MENISCI

The menisci are semilunar fibrocartilaginous discs that absorb much of the shock of weight bearing and allow seating of the femoral condyles onto the tibial condyles. The two menisci

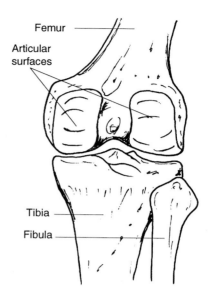

Figure 1–3 Right knee, posterior view showing bony structures.

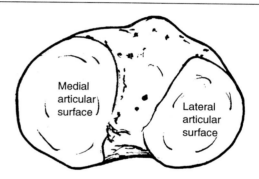

Figure 1–4 Right tibia, superior view showing articular surfaces.

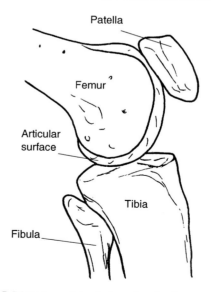

Figure 1–5 Right knee, lateral view showing bony structures.

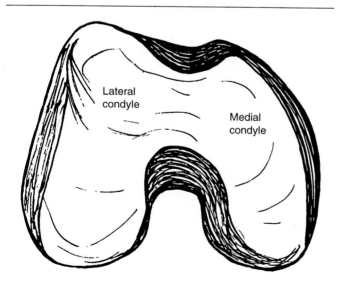

Figure 1–2 Right femur, inferior surface showing lateral and medial condyles.

are connected to each other by the anterior transverse ligament[1] (Figure 1–6).

The medial meniscus also attaches onto the anterior ridge of the tibia, called the intracondylar eminence, by the posterior horn, the capsule, and the medial collateral ligament.

The lateral meniscus is attached to the intracondylar eminence by both anterior and posterior horns, the posterior cruciate ligament, a loose connection to the capsule, and the popliteus tendon.

The intracondylar eminence attachments of the menisci as well as the cruciate attachments to the tibia are along the midline, between the femoral condyle surfaces (Figure 1–7). The cartilaginous portion (the majority) has no blood supply. The blood supply is limited to the fibrous part of the meniscus on the periphery.

Note the medial meniscus attachments on the intracondylar eminence. Its attachments posteriorly, anteriorly, and at its periphery and its greater surface allow it less movement and also leave it more susceptible to injury than its counterpart.

The intracondylar attachments of the lateral meniscus are much closer together. The minimal attachment on the periphery (anterior transverse ligament and the popliteus tendon) allows greater mobility, making the lateral meniscus less susceptible to injury.

LIGAMENTS

Cruciate Ligaments

The cruciate ligaments are named after their tibial attachments and prevent excessive shearing movement of the tibia on the femur (Figure 1–8).

The anterior cruciate inserts into the medial side of the lateral femoral condyle, preventing excessive anterior gliding of the tibia and external rotation of the tibia.

The posterior cruciate inserts into the lateral side of the medial femoral condyle, preventing excessive posterior gliding of the tibia and internal rotation of the tibia.

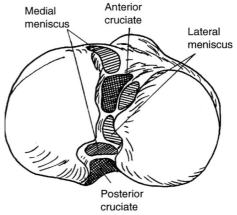

Figure 1–7 Menisci and ligament attachments.

Capsular Ligaments

The entire joint structure is secured by the capsular ligaments except above the patella and the patella itself.

The medial capsular ligaments of the knee are shown in Figure 1–9. The anterior tibial fibers traverse superiorly and anteriorly with attachments on the femur, medial meniscus, and fibers of the patella ligament.

The middle fibers are vertical, with the upper fibers securing the meniscus to the femur. The lower fibers are loosely attached to the meniscus, allowing mobility on the tibia.

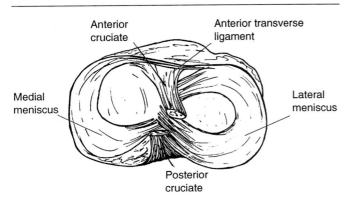

Figure 1–6 Right tibia, superior view showing major ligament attachments.

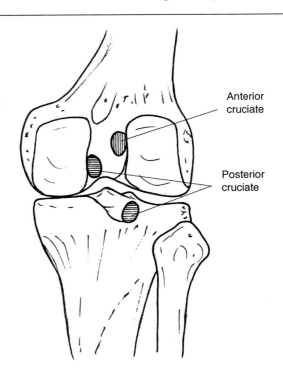

Figure 1–8 Right knee, posterior view showing cruciate ligament attachments.

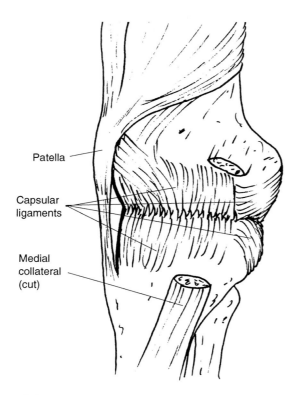

Figure 1–9 Right knee, medial view showing medial capsular ligaments.

The posterior fibers fan out and attach to the posterior part of the medial meniscus and blend with the tendon of the semimembranosus muscle inferiorly and with the gastrocnemius muscle superiorly.

The lateral capsular ligaments are shown in Figure 1–10. The anterior fibers traverse vertically, with some fibers being attached on the patella. Other fibers blend in with those from the vastus lateralis and the vastus medialis muscles. The upper portion receives fibers from the retinaculum of the vastus lateralis muscle, and the lower portion receives fibers from the iliotibial tract.

The middle fibers originate above the origin of the popliteus muscle, covering it, and attach on the lateral tibial condyle and on the anterior capsular ligament of the fibula.

The posterior fibers run vertically from the femur to the tibia and blend with the origins of the gastrocnemius muscle (Figure 1–11). It is strengthened centrally by the oblique popliteal ligament. Laterally it blends with the lateral collateral ligament.

Medially, a thickening of the capsule may be regarded as a deep component of the medial collateral ligament.

The oblique popliteal ligament is an expansion of the semimembranosus tendon and passes upward and laterally, attaching to the lateral condyle of the femur.

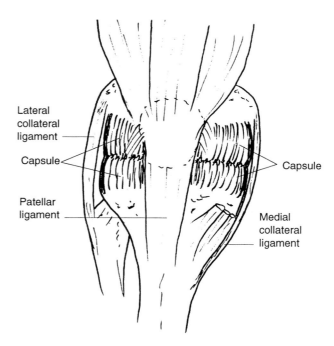

Figure 1–10 Right knee, anterior view showing lateral capsular ligaments.

The arcuate popliteal ligament arises from the fibula head in a Y shape, with some fibers attaching to the popliteus muscles and most passing over it and attaching to the intercondylar area. Some fibers may attach to the lateral head of the gastrocnemius muscle.

Note the capsule fiber's attachment to the popliteus muscle.

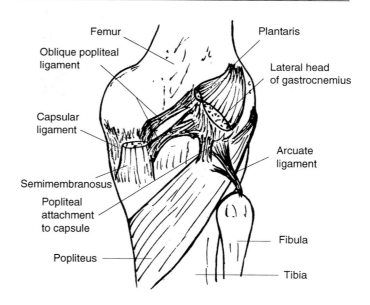

Figure 1–11 Right knee, posterior view showing capsular ligaments.

Collateral Ligaments

The medial and lateral collateral ligaments (Figure 1–12) are strong stabilizers against adduction and abduction of the tibia on the femur. They also receive help from the capsular ligaments. For the last 20° to 30° of extension the cruciate ligaments tighten, stabilizing the knee anteriorly and posteriorly and also stabilizing adduction and abduction. Therefore, testing for collateral instability should be performed with slight flexion.

Medial (Tibial) Collateral Ligament

The medial collateral ligament is superficial to the medial capsule. Its deep fibers blend with the medial capsule. The superficial fibers originate on the medial epicondyle of the femur just below the adductor tubercle. It crosses the joint slightly posterior to the midline with the fibers angled anteriorly and inserts into the shaft of the tibia below the medial condyle (Figures 1–13 and 1–14).

The deep fibers attach on the femur and the tibia above and below the joint line. Posteriorly the fibers of the medial collateral ligaments have attachments to the semimembranosus muscle, the capsule, and the medial meniscus. Several bursae are located between the medial collateral ligament, the capsule, and the meniscus.

Lateral (Fibular) Collateral Ligament

The lateral collateral ligament (Figure 1–15) originates on the lateral epicondyle of the femur superior and slightly posterior to the origin of the popliteus muscle, passing over it and inserting into the head of the fibula. Its insertion is surrounded by the biceps femoris tendon (see Figure 1–12).

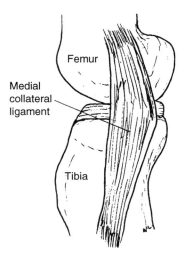

Figure 1–13 Right knee, extended, medial view showing medial collateral ligament.

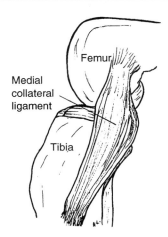

Figure 1–14 Right knee, flexed, medial view showing medial collateral ligament.

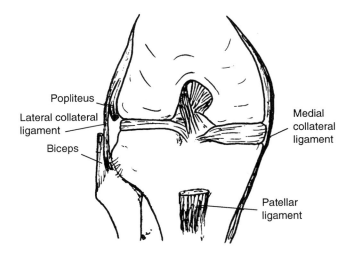

Figure 1–12 Right knee, anterior view showing medial and lateral collateral ligaments.

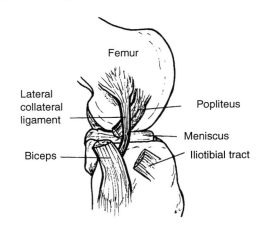

Figure 1–15 Right knee, lateral view showing collateral ligament.

Patellar Ligament

The common tendon of the quadriceps inserts into the superior border of the patella. The tendons of the vastus lateralis and vastus medialis insert on their respective sides of the patella. The superficial fibers of the tendons encompass the patella and blend with the patellar ligament. The patellar ligament originates above on the apex and sides of the patella and inserts below into the tibial tuberosity (Figure 1–16).

The ligaments, menisci, and muscle attachments on the tibial surface depicted in Figure 1–17 show their unique relationships.

BURSAE

- Anterior (Figure 1–18)

  1. The suprapatellar bursa is between the femur and the quadriceps tendon.
  2. The prepatellar (subcutaneous) bursa is between the skin and the patella. This bursa is involved in the so-called housemaid's knee.
  3. The superficial infrapatellar bursa is between the skin and the patellar ligament.
  4. The deep infrapatellar bursa is between the upper tibia and the patellar ligament.[2]

- Medial (Figures 1–18 and 1–19)

  1. One is between the gastrocnemius muscle and the capsule.

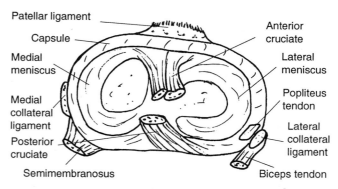
Figure 1–17 Right tibia articular surface.

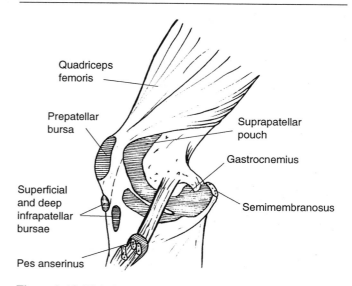
Figure 1–18 Right knee, medial view showing bursae.

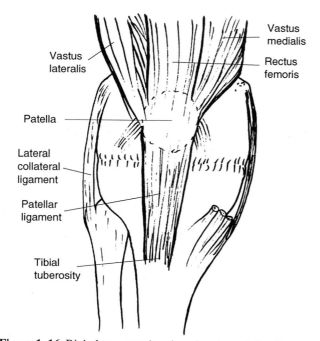
Figure 1–16 Right knee, anterior view showing patellar ligament.

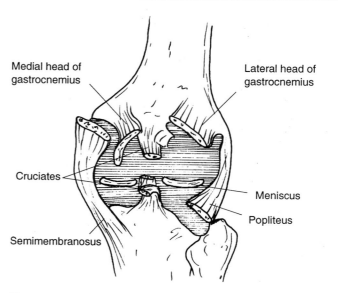
Figure 1–19 Right knee, posterior view showing bursae.

2. One is between the medial collateral ligament and the pes anserinus (attachment of the sartorius, gracilis, and semitendinosus muscles).
3. Several are between the expanse of the medial collateral ligament and the femur, meniscus, tibia, capsule, and semimembranosus muscle.
4. One is between the semimembranosus, the gastrocnemius, and the condyle of the tibia. Occasionally it is connected with the capsule. Inflammation and effusion of this bursa (bursitis) is commonly referred to as Baker's cyst.

- Lateral (Figure 1–19)
  1. One is between the popliteus muscle and the lateral condyle of the femur. This bursa usually communicates with the capsule.
  2. One is between the popliteus and the lateral collateral ligament.
  3. One is between the lateral collateral ligament and the biceps femoris tendon (not shown).
  4. One is between the capsule and the lateral head of the gastrocnemius.

MUSCLE ATTACHMENTS

Figure 1–20 is an anterior view of the right knee showing the relative positions of the quadriceps muscles (except the vastus intermedialis, which is deep to the rectus) and their convergence into the quadriceps tendon. Note that the lower fibers of the vastus medialis originate lower than those of the vastus lateralis and traverse at an oblique angle to the patella. The iliotibial tract inserts on the anterior portion of the lateral tibial condyle.

The sartorius, gracilis, and semitendinosus muscles attach on the tibia below the medial condyle on the anteromedial surface (pes anserinus; Figure 1–21).

The semimembranosus (Figure 1–22) lies deep to the semitendinosus and inserts above it on the posterior tibial condyle. The medial head of the gastrocnemius passes lateral to both hamstring muscles and inserts into the posterior surface of the medial condyle of the femur.

The vastus medialis muscle (Figure 1–22) originates on the medial edge of the posterior surface of the femur. Some fibers insert into the common quadriceps tendon and the medial border of the patella. This muscle also gives off fibers to the capsule. Note that the distal oblique fibers originate just proximal to the adductor tubercle and provide medial stability to the patella.

The popliteal fossa (Figure 1–22) is formed medially by the three pes anserinus muscles and the semimembranosus. Its superior and lateral borders are formed by the tendons of biceps femoris. Inferiorly it is formed by the two heads of the gastrocnemius and plantaris muscles.

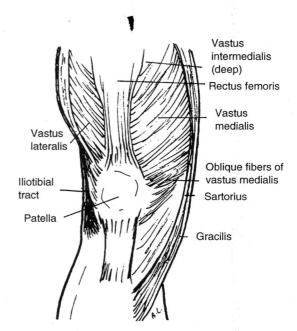

Figure 1–20 Right knee, anterior view showing muscle attachments.

The angle of the vastus lateralis from its origin to its insertion into the patella is approximately 30° (compared to 55° for the vastus medialis; Figures 1–23 and 1–24).

The biceps femoris inserts into the fibula head by two bands surrounding the insertion of the lateral collateral ligament.

The iliotibial tract is a thick band of fasciae on the lateral thigh originating with the insertions of the gluteus maximums and the tensor fascia lata muscles. As it approaches the knee it

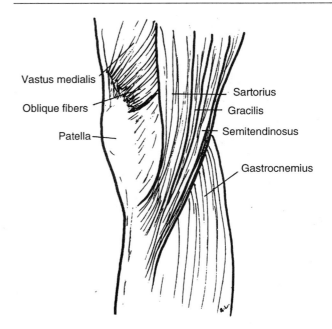

Figure 1–21 Right knee, medial view showing muscle attachments.

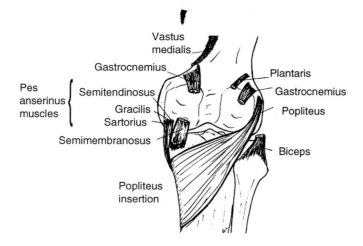

Figure 1–22 Right knee, posterior view showing muscle attachments.

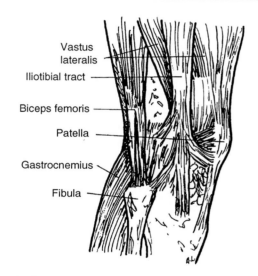

Figure 1–23 Right knee, lateral view showing muscle attachments.

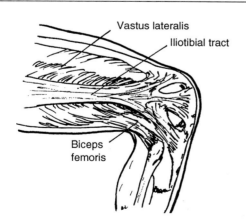

Figure 1–24 Right knee, flexed, lateral view showing muscle attachments.

spreads out, attaching to the expansion from the vastus lateralis muscle and to all the exposed bone segments of the knee, including the fibula. Its greatest attachment is to the tubercle on the anterior surface of the lateral tibial condyle.

FUNCTIONAL ANATOMY

Flexion

Muscles

Active flexion (movement produced by the patient) of the knee with the hip extended usually will not exceed 120°. This is due to the restraint of the rectus femoris muscles and the loss of hamstring efficiency[3] (Figure 1–25). Active flexion may reach 140° with the hip flexed[3] (Figure 1–26).

Active flexion normally produces movement of the heel toward the ischial tuberosity. The most common deviation from the normal is the heel retracting medial to the tuberosity[4,5] (Figure 1–27). This is usually due to a lateral rotation fixation of the tibia on the femur or an imbalance of the muscles. The biceps and/or iliotibial tract may be hypertonic, or the popliteus and/or medial hamstrings may be weak (by comparison).

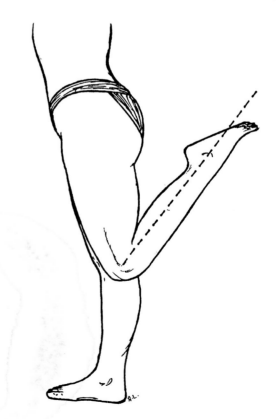

Figure 1–25 Active flexion of the knee to 120°.

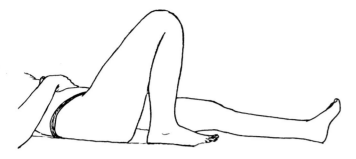

Figure 1–26 Active flexion of the knee with the hip flexed.

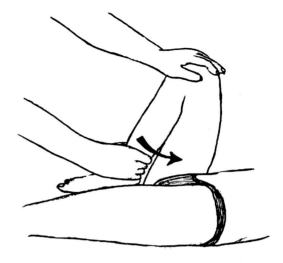

Figure 1–28 Passive flexion of the knee.

Passive flexion (movement produced by the examiner) may attain 160° and may allow the heel to touch the buttocks in line with the ischial tuberosity[3] (Figure 1–28).

Active flexion from full extension begins with medial (internal) rotation of the tibia initiated by contraction of the popliteus muscle.[6]

The most powerful flexors of the knee are the hamstrings: biceps femoris, semimembranosus, and semitendinosus (Figure 1–29). Flexion is initiated by the popliteus muscle (not shown). All the hamstring muscles cross two joints; therefore, they affect both and are affected by both. Their action on the knee is stronger with the hip flexed than with the hip extended.

Note the origin of the biceps. Along with the other hamstring muscles, it attaches to the ischial tuberosity. It also

originates some fibers on the sacrotuberous ligament,[1] giving it influence on the sacroiliac joint and thus affecting the entire posture. The short head of the biceps originates on the posterior surface of the femur between the adductor magnus and the vastus lateralis. It then joins the long head to form the biceps tendon, inserting into the head of the fibula.

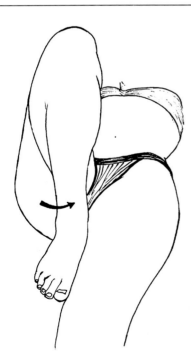

Figure 1–27 Active flexion of the knee with the heel medial.

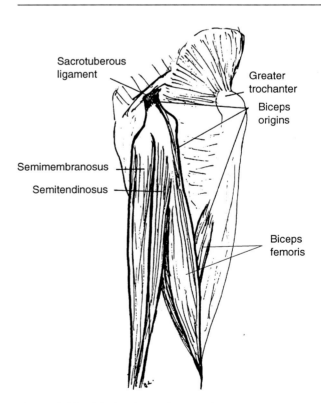

Figure 1–29 Right leg, hamstring muscles.

The sartorius and gracilis muscles each contribute to flexion and medial rotation of the tibia (Figure 1–30). The sartorius with its origin on the anterosuperior iliac spine also assists in flexion of the hip joint. The gracilis with its origin on the pubis is a strong flexor of the knee and assists in adduction of the hip.[1,6]

The gastrocnemius muscle assists in flexion. The greatest effect is with the ankle dorsiflexed. The plantaris muscle has a similar action, but its size precludes any great contribution to flexion.

Medial Meniscus

During flexion, tibial contact with the femur moves posteriorly[6] (Figure 1–31). The medial meniscus' contact with the articular surface of the femoral condyle and its attachment to the rim of the tibial condyle allow distortion to occur and create susceptibility to injury.

In active flexion, the posterior horn is pulled posteriorly by the semimembranosus muscle, while the anterior horn is retained by its attachments and is pulled anteriorly by fibers attached to the anterior cruciate ligament.

In passive flexion, the posterior horn is retained anteriorly without the posterior pull of the semimembranosus muscle.

Lateral Meniscus

In flexion, the lateral meniscus, like the medial meniscus, moves posterior. The anterior horn attachment on the intercondylar eminence rather than on the rim of the tibia allows

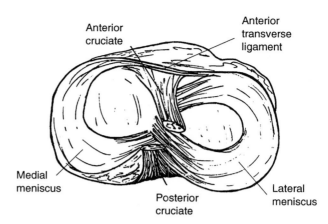

Figure 1–31 Right tibia, superior view showing major ligament attachments.

greater mobility during movement. In flexion the popliteus muscle pulls the lateral meniscus posteriorly while moving the posterior capsule, preventing entrapment between the femur and the tibia.

Transverse (Anterior) Ligament

During flexion the patella moves inferiorly and, through its attachment, allows the transverse ligament to move posteriorly (Figure 1–31). This allows some posterior movement of the menisci yet restrains movement to either side from the midline.

Cruciate Ligaments

The anterior cruciate originates on the anterior intercondylar area of the tibia and traverses posteriorly, superiorly, and laterally with the posterior attachment on the medial side of the lateral femoral condyle (Figure 1–31). During flexion the ligament lies between the femoral condyles and between the intercondylar eminences of the tibia. At 90° of flexion the anterior cruciate lies horizontally, and in full flexion the fibers are relaxed.

The posterior cruciate originates on the posterior intercondylar area of the tibia and the lateral meniscus (Figures 1–32 and 1–33). It passes anteriorly, superiorly, and medially to attach on the lateral surface of the medial condyle of the femur. It is much shorter than the anterior cruciate. During flexion it becomes almost vertical.

Extension

Normal active extension goes slightly beyond 0°, allowing approximately 5° to 10° of hyperextension (Figure 1–34). The 5° to 10° of hyperextension allows erect standing without quadriceps function. Farther extension is prevented by the capsular and other posterior ligaments as well as by the normal muscle tone of the popliteus.

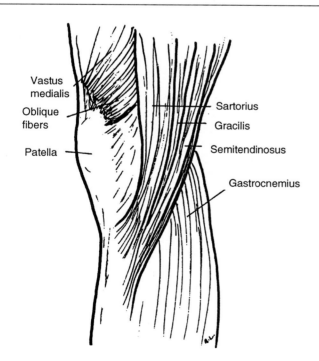

Figure 1–30 Right knee, medial view showing muscle attachments.

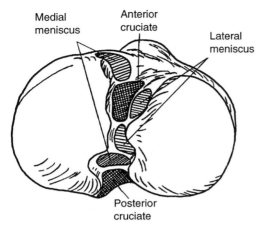

Figure 1–32 Menisci and ligament attachments.

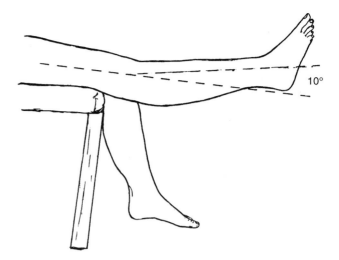

Figure 1–34 Right knee, normal hyperextension.

The primary extensors are the rectus femoris, vastus intermedialis, vastus medialis, and vastus lateralis (quadriceps femoris; Figure 1–35). They are assisted by the action of the tensor fascia lata and gluteus maximus muscles through the iliotibial tract.

The extensors are approximately three times stronger than the flexors, counteracting gravity and providing mediolateral stability. They also act as decelerators in changes of gait and in actions such as walking downhill or abrupt landing after a jump.

The vastus intermedialis is the deepest of the muscles, originating on the anterior and lateral surface of the femur.

The rectus femoris originates with two heads on the anteroinferior iliac spine and the groove above the acetabulum and is the only one of the quadriceps to cross two joints. Its actions upon the knee are strongest with the hip extended.

The vastus lateralis originates under the greater trochanter and the lateral aspect of the posterior surface of the femur along the linea aspera femoris and the gluteal tuberosity (Figure 1–36).

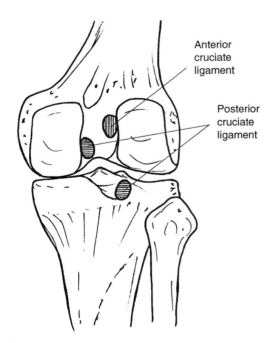

Figure 1–33 Right knee, posterior view showing cruciate ligament attachments.

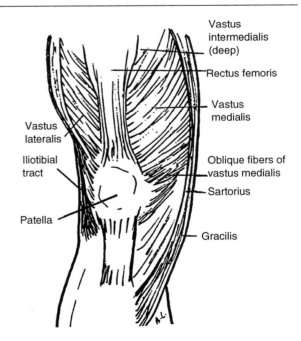

Figure 1–35 Right knee, anterior view showing muscle attachments.

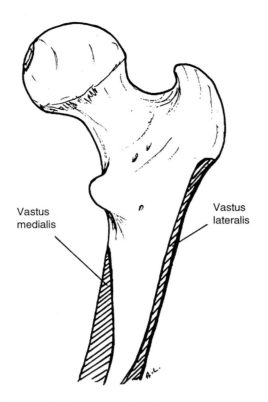

Vastus
medialis

Vastus
lateralis

Figure 1–36 Right femur, posterior view.

The vastus medialis originates along the medial aspect of the posterior femur with the lowest fibers almost horizontal to the upper border of the patella.

The articularis genus is a small muscle below the rectus femoris that originates on the anterior surface of the femur. It often blends with the vastus intermedialis muscle. It elevates the synovial membrane (lining of the capsule) during extension.

Some fibers of the vastus medialis attach to the capsular ligaments and the medial condyle of the tibia. Fibers from the vastus lateralis attach to the capsular ligaments, the lateral condyle of the tibia, and the iliotibial tract.

The quadriceps muscles attach to the common quadriceps tendon, which in turn encompasses the patella and passes through the patellar ligament to the tibia.

The tensor fascia lata, acting upon the iliotibial tract, assists in extension with the hip extended. Quadriceps function is strongest with the hip straight or in extension, allowing the greatest response by the rectus femoris muscle.

Action of the rectus femoris and vastus intermedialis extends the knee. The vastus medialis and vastus lateralis provide extension strength and retain the patella in its articular groove. Through their capsular, iliotibial, and tibial attachments, they also provide stabilization to the knee during extension movement.

Electromyographic studies show that not all the muscles perform simultaneously but vary from phase to phase during extension. It is generally accepted that the vastus medialis muscle has minimal function except for the last 15° to 20° of extension. It has been my experience that it is of great importance during the entire movement from extreme flexion to hyperextension. These findings will be discussed in Chapter 6.

As the patella is pulled superiorly during extension, its ligamental fibers' attachment to the anterior transverse ligament pulls it forward, and thus the menisci are pulled forward (Figure 1-37).[6]

Moving from flexion to extension, upon reaching approximately 10° to 20° the lateral condyle ceases movement. The balance of extension consists of the tibia pivoting on the lateral femoral condyle and the medial condyle of the tibia moving anteriorly. The additional anterior movement of the medial tibial condyle (lateral rotation) tightens the cruciate and collateral ligaments with a screw-home effect, stabilizing the knee in extension and normal hyperextension.

Rotation

The screw-home effect stabilizes the knee and prevents mediolateral movement. At the same time it locks the tibia in lateral rotation; the tibia is limited and secured by the ligaments and the intercondylar eminence. In normal hyperextension, rotation is prevented in either direction.

Passive movement of the knee from hyperextension to neutral (0° of extension) unlocks the screw-home effect. It also allows medial rotation of the tibia back into neutral, allowing approximately 10° of lateral rotation and 5° of medial rotation of the tibia. As the knee flexes further, the range of rotary motion increases, with the greatest range occurring at 100°. At 100° of flexion, lateral rotation is approximately 15° and me-

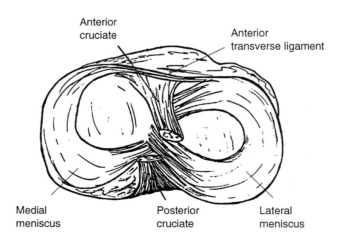

Anterior
cruciate

Anterior
transverse ligament

Medial
meniscus

Posterior
cruciate

Lateral
meniscus

Figure 1–37 Right tibia, superior view showing major ligament attachments.

dial rotation approximately 10°. In complete flexion, lateral rotation is restricted while medial rotation remains approximately 10°.

During rotation the menisci distort with the femur; thus, as lateral rotation of the tibia occurs, the lateral meniscus is pulled toward the anterior tibial condyle while the medial meniscus is drawn posteriorly. The reverse occurs during medial rotation.

Medial (internal) rotation of the foot, ankle, and tibia with the knee at 90° of flexion will be approximately 30° (Figure 1–38); lateral (external) rotation will be approximately 40° (Figure 1–39). Passive rotation may increase both by approximately 5°. Ligament laxity varies from individual to individual; therefore, always compare to the well knee and to the flexibility of the other main joints of the body.

The primary medial rotators, the popliteus and medial hamstrings (Figure 1–40), are assisted by the sartorius and gracilis. They are also assisted by some fibers of the vastus medialis and, with the ankle dorsiflexed, the medial head of the gastrocnemius.

The primary lateral rotators are the biceps femoris, the tensor fascia lata (iliotibial tract), and the gluteus maximus

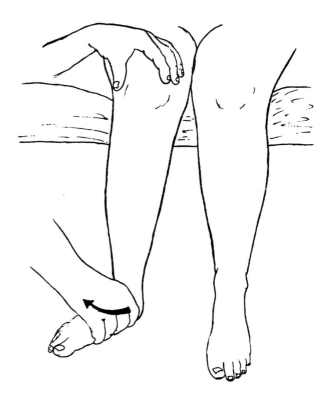

Figure 1–39 Lateral rotation of the foot, ankle, and tibia to 40° with the knee flexed at 90°.

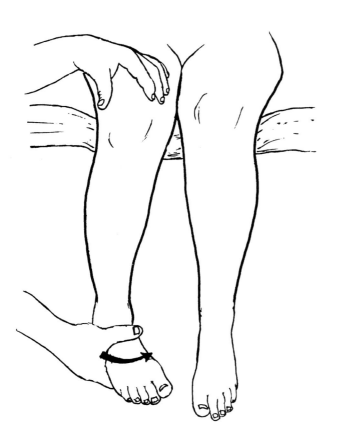

Figure 1–38 Medial rotation of the foot, ankle, and tibia to 30° with the knee flexed at 90°.

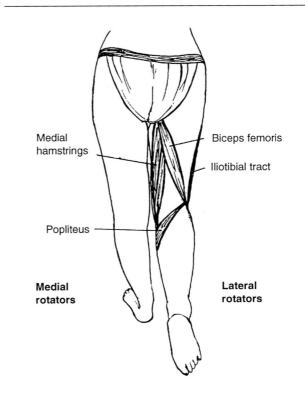

Figure 1–40 Rotators of the right tibia.

through the iliotibial tract. With the ankle dorsiflexed, the lateral head of the gastrocnemius assists lateral rotation.

Fibula-Tibia Articulation

Although the fibula is not part of the knee proper, it plays an important part in knee function. The fibula's ligamental attachments on the femur (lateral collateral ligament), the knee capsule, and the tibia may affect knee function.

Movement of the fibula on the tibia is governed by the fibula's location on the posterolateral surface of the tibia as the condyle begins to narrow and by its muscle attachments. Movements of the proximal end of the fibula are:

1. anteroinferior, by actions of the peroneus longus and extensor digitorum longus muscles
2. superior, by action of the biceps femoris with the knee extended
3. superoposterior, by action of the biceps, depending on the degree of flexion (past 90° the movement is posterior)
4. inferior, by action of the flexor hallucis longus and extensor digitorum longus muscles

REFERENCES

1. Warwick R, Williams P. *Gray's Anatomy*. 35th British ed. Philadelphia: Saunders; 1973.
2. McMinn RM, Hutchings RT. *Color Atlas of Human Anatomy*. Chicago: Year Book Medical; 1977.
3. Hoppenfeld S. *Physical Examination of the Spine and Extremities*. New York: Appleton-Century-Crofts; 1976.
4. Kapandji IA. *The Physiology of the Joints*. New York: Churchill Livingstone; 1977. Baltimore: Williams & Wilkins; 1986;1 and 2.
5. Yochum T. *Essentials of Skeletal Radiology*. Baltimore: Williams & Wilkins; 1986;1 and 2.
6. Turek SL. *Orthopaedics, Principles and Their Application*. Philadelphia: Lippincott; 1967.

HISTORY

Before examination, a thorough history is necessary to enable the examiner to continue in a logical manner. The consistency of examination findings with the history is important in arriving at a proper treatment program.

Occupation

Individuals in occupations involving the use of the knees, such as cement masons, carpet layers, and baseball catchers, have stresses unique to their professions that must be considered. Individuals with sedentary occupations during the week who participate in weekend activities involving knee stress, such as roofing, cement work, baseball, and skiing, are more susceptible to injury.

Has there been a change in the patient's routine recently?

Recreation

Has the patient started any new recreation that may be a factor?

Exercise

Has the patient started, or changed, an exercise program?

Sleep Position

Whether the patient presents with a knee, low back, or cervical spine problem, it is important to investigate the posture of sleep. Remaining in the wrong position for 5 to 8 hours each night will produce muscle imbalances that contribute to, or cause, problems involving the knee.

Most prone sleepers are susceptible because:

- the head is turned to one side, stretching one group of cervical muscles while allowing the opposite group to contract because the origin is held closer to the insertion
- if the head turns to the left, the left femur must rotate laterally with the foot to the left and the knee bent and with the tibia laterally rotated
- the right rotates medially
- to remain in this position, the entire pelvis must rotate anteriorly, increasing the lumbar curve

Other prone sleepers may lie with both feet in one direction or with each foot rotated laterally and both arms stretched over the head.

All the above produce distortions that the alert observer may use in establishing the correct treatment program. Sometimes questioning of the spouse is necessary to gather this information.

Preexisting Conditions

Any trauma before the onset of symptoms? What other problems have existed that required treatment by a health professional?

Onset

Gradual

When did the symptoms *first* appear? When did the symptoms increase sufficiently for the patient to seek help? Was there a change in activity before the onset of symptoms?

Sudden

When did the symptoms suddenly appear, and was there a reason to the patient's knowledge?

If the patient received a blow, by what object? From what direction? How hard? Was the knee straight or bent? Was the foot planted? Was there a "pop"? Was there immediate disability? Was there immediate pain? Was there swelling, and if so, how soon after the trauma?

If caused by abnormal body movement, skiing? If so, exactly what was the position of the ski in relationship to the body? What direction was the momentum? In what direction did the knee go? Was there a "pop"? Did the patient feel the knee "give way"?

If caused by a slip and fall, on which foot was traction lost? Was the loss of control the *result* of knee pain, or was the knee pain the result of the injury? Did the patient break the fall? If so, with what part of the body? What part (or parts) did the patient land on?

OBSERVATION

Observation should begin, if possible, with the patient walking into the examination room, continue while the patient is sitting during the history, follow the patient's movement from the chair, and include gowning or undressing. Any abnormal gait, placement of the feet, obvious discomfort, and/or difficulty in sitting or rising should be noted.

To recognize abnormal sitting, standing posture, or movements, it is necessary to observe many patients without symptoms and to have an understanding of what normal is. Knowledge of what muscles and structures are involved in normal movement allows the observer to focus on the problem efficiently.

The nonambulatory patient must be examined in a non–weight-bearing position, preferably supine (to be discussed later). For the purposes of this text, the examination procedures are based on the ambulatory patient in the order used by the author. The text does not necessarily follow the rigid divisions of observation, palpation, orthopedic testing, muscle testing, and so forth.

Standing

With the patient gowned or undressed sufficiently to observe the entire body, begin the examination in the erect posture.

Instruct the patient to stand with the feet even but not touching. Make sure the knees do not touch (some obese patients with extreme valgus knees or patients with overdeveloped thigh muscles may find it necessary to stand with the feet wider apart). With this instruction, the patient will usually assume the foot placement that habit patterns allow. Any unilat-

eral rotation of the foot should be noted as a part of the patient's habit pattern. If unilateral rotation is found, have the patient correct the stance with each foot in 5° to 10° of lateral rotation.

Toeing out (Figure 2–1) is common in anatomic short leg, hip problems (including lateral rotation from prone sleeping), and other postural faults as well as in knee problems.

Patients who automatically stand toeing out may resist placing the feet in the correct position. Whether toeing out is a result of other postural faults or the cause of postural faults has yet to be determined. Patients will feel uncomfortable when instructed to place the feet correctly.

This indicates that the patient's body has compensated for the abnormality and automatically assumes the position best suited to respond to the command to stand erect. Correction of the foot placement reveals the true distortion pattern if one exists.

To continue the examination without correcting the foot placement would be a mistake. This also applies to positioning for standing X-rays. By insisting upon the correct position, the observer has the opportunity to observe the true distortions from the foot up. If films are provided of the standing lumbosacral spine, the appearance of the lesser trochanter and the greater trochanter–femur head distance will give a clue to whether the foot placement was correct.

If possible, the patient should maintain the erect posture for at least 1 full minute. It takes approximately 1 minute for the postural muscles to allow the normal posture to be assumed.

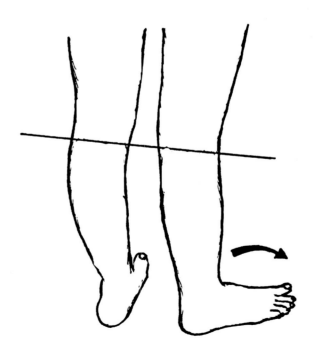

Figure 2–1 Lateral rotation.

During the interval, any movement of the body to adapt to the position should be noted.

Always compare the involved knee with the uninvolved one.

Posterior Observation

With the patient maintaining the erect posture, observation of the body may begin with the feet. With some patients it is difficult to maintain the posture; they may turn around to ask a question or respond to a question. The patient must be reminded to keep looking straight forward without any conscious movement.

Postural faults from a tilted head, high shoulder, and spinal distortions may be either contributing to or caused by a lower extremity problem. Any distortion below the iliac crest must be considered directly involved with the knee problem. In chronic knee problems, the distortion may be the cause of knee symptoms. Trauma to the knee may be the cause of the distortion. All the distortions must be investigated to achieve success.

The logical approach to examining any structure is to start with the base. Any imbalance will produce a reaction of the structures above to enable the body to compensate and remain standing.

Pronation of the Calcaneus

Any disturbance of the normal posture of the foot that interferes with the distance from floor to tibia will result in an apparent (physiologic or functional) short leg. One of the most common causes is pronation of the calcaneus.

With pronation of the calcaneus, a leg length inequality may exist (Figure 2–2). If pronation of the forefoot occurs with the calcaneus not involved, no leg length inequality will exist. A unilateral pronated foot without trauma usually indicates poor body mechanics, and the reason must be investigated.

Pronation is a common finding in the laterally rotated femur, the anatomically short leg, and the valgus knee. The examiner must keep in mind that with any of the above pronation may or may not involve the calcaneus.

Knee Fold Height

Compare the knee fold height. With both feet the same, a low knee fold may indicate a possible anatomically short tibia (Figure 2–3).

Unilateral Flexion-Extension of the Knee

Compare flexion-extension of the knees. Unilateral flexion (Figure 2–4) may indicate:

- chronic flexion of an anatomically long leg (a reaction to the attempt to level the pelvis)

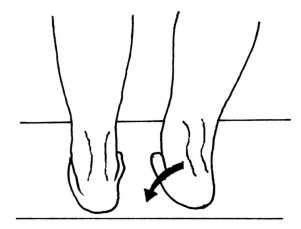

Figure 2–2 Pronated right foot.

- the inability to bear weight without pain (ask the patient to shift weight to the flexed side to obtain a possible reaction)
- pelvis distortion, for whatever reason, making it necessary to flex one knee to maintain posture
- possible bilateral genu recurvatum with the patient unable to extend the knee fully on one side

Genu recurvatum is found more often in women and individuals with lax ligaments.[1] It may be congenital or acquired from injury to the musculature causing equinus deformity of the foot.[2] The possibility exists that a patient with what may

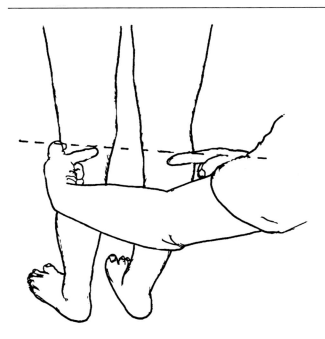

Figure 2–3 Palpation for knee fold height.

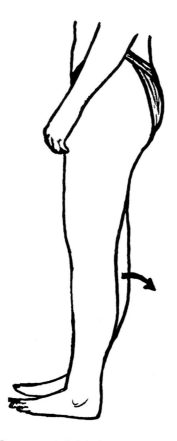

Figure 2–4 Hyperextended right knee.

appear to be a unilateral hyperextended knee may be a patient with genu recurvatum (hyperextended knees) who has a *flexed* knee, which would of course appear more normal. It has been the author's experience that genu recurvatum usually is bilateral. It usually is symptom-free, and when the popliteus muscle is tested properly it may be normal unless affected by recent injury.

Unilateral hyperextension may indicate:

- damaged ligaments
- a weakened popliteus muscle
- gallbladder dysfunction (see Appendix A)
- pelvic distortion, for whatever reason, making it necessary to flex both knees to maintain the erect posture

Observe for the following:

- edema
- abnormal muscle tone or atrophy. Compare to the asymptomatic knee. While comparing, the examiner must keep in mind that what may appear as a lack of muscle tone or an abnormal contraction may be a result of the inability to stand without pain. Abnormal tone or atrophy may also be affected by other postural consider-

ations. Always compare with the non–weight-bearing findings.

- abnormal medial deviation (valgus) or lateral deviation (varus) of the knee
- varicosities, abrasions, or discolorations

Palpate for possible alterations of skin temperature.

Anterior Observation

Valgus Knee

A valgus condition of the knee (knock knees; Figure 2–5) may be an overall postural fault (bilateral) or an imbalance that has produced a unilateral valgus condition (discussed in Chapter 6).

Varus Knee

A varus knee (bowlegs; Figure 2–6) may be congenital or postural; it is believed to be caused by the infant's lying in the

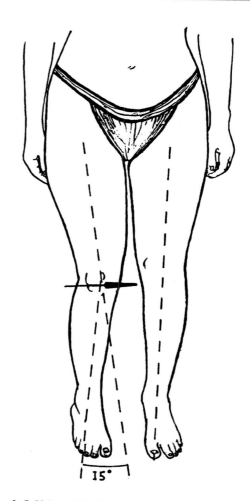

Figure 2–5 Valgus right knee.

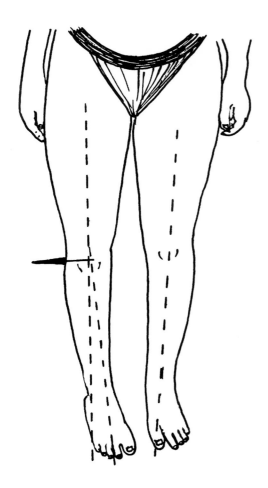

Figure 2–6 Varus right knee.

prone position with the thighs abducted and the toes turned inward.[2] Adolescent varus usually makes its appearance between 6 and 12 years of age.[2]

Observe the feet for any obvious stress. Look for disturbances in the forefoot–hindfoot relationship compared with the other foot. Whiteness and obvious gripping of the floor with the toes is a sign of disturbance in weight bearing.

Ask the patient to relate where he or she feels the body weight on the feet as the posture is maintained. In the normal body with a normal foot, the patient should not be able to relate any specific area. Usually if a general area such as the heel or front of one foot is sensed by the patient, it would indicate a postural distortion elsewhere in the body. If the weight is felt specifically on an area such as "under my big toe," it usually indicates a fixation or other disturbance in the foot itself.

Look for obvious tibial rotation that may be associated with a fixation of the knee, pronated foot, valgus knee, or hyperextension.

Height of the patella is important. If the low side corresponds with a low knee fold finding without a pronated foot,

an anatomic short tibia may be expected. A finding of a hypertonic quadriceps musculature would be significant on the high patella side. In the erect posture, the relaxed, slightly hyperextended knee needs little quadriceps function.

Look for any other abnormal muscle contractions and/or atrophy. Atrophy of the oblique fibers of the vastus medialis muscle (VMO) occurs rapidly after injury.

Note any apparent edema above, below, or to the sides of the patella. Observation should include a search for scars of old injuries and/or surgeries that the patient failed to reveal during the history.

Always compare the upright findings with the non–weight-bearing ones.

Functional Testing

The ambulatory patient may be asked to perform the following procedures while the examiner observes any abnormal motion or obvious distress. Observation is important because some patients are reluctant to report pain or difficulty during the performance. If movement cannot be accomplished completely, at what point was it necessary to stop? If it becomes necessary to stop, it is important to know whether it was from pain or just the inability to continue because of weakness.

The following tests for the seemingly simple task of rising from sitting to standing and lowering from standing to sitting have been used by the author for many years. Their use, with proper observation, often reveals many obvious faults, known or unknown to the patient.

Erect Examination

Have the patient, with the feet even, sit down on a normal chair or stool (16 to 18 in from the floor) without use of the hands (Figure 2–7).

Observe for smoothness of movement or lack of it. Movement should not consist of "letting go" and dropping into the chair rapidly.

Look for hesitation and/or apprehension during the movement.

Observe the knees during the movement for abnormal shifting medially or laterally. Lateral movement of the knee during the sitting down movement indicates a dependence on the lateral stabilizers and possible problems on the medial side of the knee. Lateral movement is also a method of compensating for a back problem and may be used to allow the back to remain rigid during the process of sitting down. Medial movement of the knee during the sitting process may also be used to compensate for a back problem or a dependence on the medial knee stabilizers.

Have the patient, with the feet even and the knees flexed to 90°, rise to standing *without use of the hands*. From behind the patient, observe the movements of the torso, buttocks, and knees during the attempt.

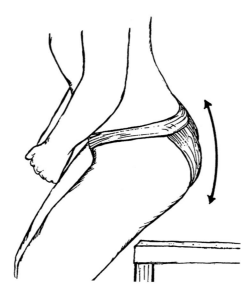

Figure 2–7 Sitting or rising without use of the hands.

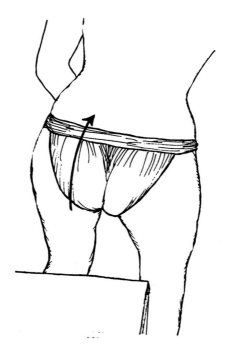

Figure 2–8 Rising to standing with most of the weight on the right leg.

If no abnormal movement occurs, have the patient move the feet forward 3 to 5 in and repeat (this requires greater effort).

If rising cannot be performed, have the patient move the feet 3 to 5 in posterior of 90°. This makes it easier to rise; if possible, observe the movement.

Have the patient, with the feet even, rise to standing with 80% to 85% of the weight on one foot, then on the opposite foot (Figure 2–8). This requires greater effort with dependence on only one knee and may reveal lumbar and/or sacroiliac problems that may or may not be associated with the knee problem. The patient may be unable to rise or may have to exaggerate pelvic movement to one side or the other with obvious abnormal movement.

Have the patient, while holding onto a desk or table, attempt a squat (Figure 2–9).

Look at the attempt for hesitation, apprehension, smoothness of movement, or abnormal movements of the knee and/or body. If the squat cannot be completed, note the point at which movement becomes limited and whether there is pain associated with it. The limitation of movement may be compared later with range of motion tests in the non–weight-bearing supine position. Have the patient identify the exact location of the pain if possible.

Watch the attempt to stand erect for the same abnormalities as noted above and the degree of flexion at which movement becomes painful, is difficult to perform, or is not possible to continue.

Supine Examination

Close observation during movement from standing to achieve the supine posture may verify a finding already identi-

fied as a possibility and may help in finding other problems. In some cases of malingering, it may reveal an ability to function that was claimed as not possible during functional testing.

Look carefully at *both* legs for obvious atrophy, muscle contractions, edema, and inability to straighten the knee. If at-

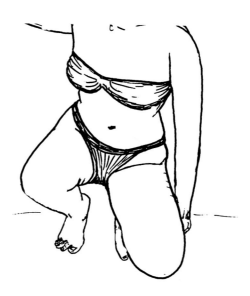

Figure 2–9 Squatting.

rophy is suspected, measure the thighs 3 in above the patella and compare. Absence of the normal hollow between the vastus medialis and the patella would indicate possible edema.

The most common area to atrophy is the oblique fibers of the vastus medialis muscle (Figure 2–10). Atrophy of these occurs soon after injury or surgery to the medial knee. A lack of substance may have been present before the injury or surgery and, if so, would have been at the least a contributing factor.

Look at the legs in the resting position and again when lifting the legs to check for possible hyperextension. Atrophy may appear nearly normal at first glance and be overlooked, yet with the legs suspended and relaxed the bulk will appear diminished.

Palpation of the Quadriceps Femoris

Careful palpation of the quadriceps while comparing with its opposite may reveal fiber reactions (trigger points), muscle contractions, lack of tone, or areas of possible muscle tear (Figure 2–11).

After examining the muscle bulk, locate the insertion of the oblique fibers of the vastus medialis on the patella. To identify those fibers in the extended knee, have the patient contract the quadriceps several times while palpating the medial border of the patella. The fibers may be traced almost horizontally under the sartorius and to their origin on the posterior edge of the medial femur just above the adductor tubercle.

Palpate around the patella edge for pain, edema, and increase in temperature (Figure 2–12).

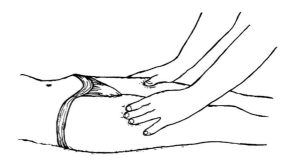

Figure 2–11 Palpation of the quadriceps femoris.

To test for pain and edema under the patella, push the patella posteriorly into the trochlear groove, which will displace excess fluid from underneath (Figure 2–13). Quick release of the patella permits the return of the fluid and "floating" of the patella. With edema, the normal dimpling of the tissue medial and slightly proximal to the patella will be missing.

If pain is present on pushing the patella into the groove, have the patient contract the quadriceps while applying pressure. Increased pain may indicate a direct injury to the anterior condyle (if hit with the knee flexed) or a degenerative condition involving the trochlear groove and/or the patella.

With a thumb web, contact the patella and push inferiorly (Figure 2–14). Resistance would indicate a possible contracture of the quadriceps femoris muscles.

Push the patella proximally, testing for mobility and pain. If pain is present in a young patient, consider Osgood-Schlatter

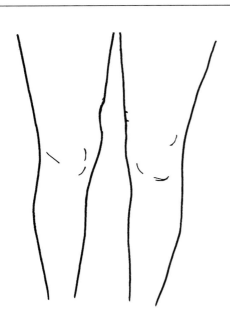

Figure 2–10 Vastus medialis oblique fiber atrophy.

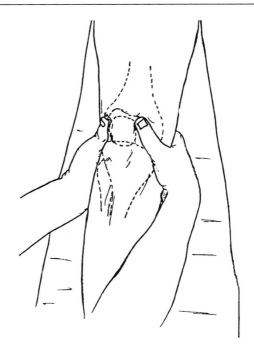

Figure 2–12 Right knee, palpation around the patella.

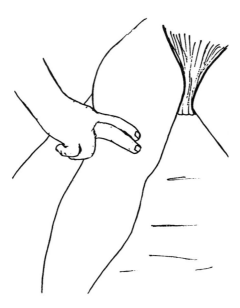

Figure 2–13 Right knee, palpation for edema and pain.

disease (osteochondritis of the tibial tubercle). Larsen-Johansson disease (osteochondritis of the patella, usually the inferior pole) will also produce pain.

Patellar Ligament

With any trauma case, direct injury to the patella, patellar ligament, and tibial tubercle must be considered.

Palpate the entire extent of the ligament for areas of reported pain. Palpate carefully for any interruption of the normal vertical fibers (Figure 2–15).

Tibial Tubercle

Palpate around the entire tubercle, again observing for areas of reported pain or abnormality (Figure 2–16).

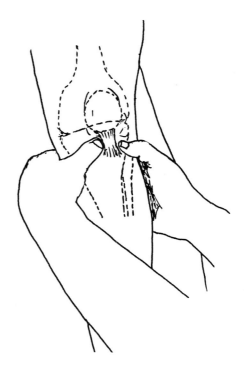

Figure 2–15 Palpation of the patellar-tibial ligament.

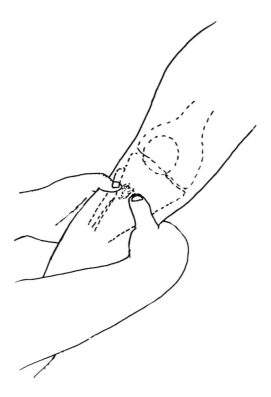

Figure 2–16 Palpation of the tibial tubercle.

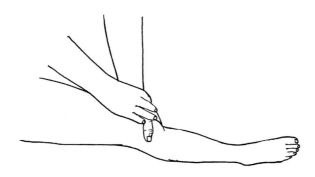

Figure 2–14 Palpation for tight quadriceps femoris.

Medial Displacement of the Patella

Medial displacement or increased mobility seldom occurs because of the lack of stressors to produce it (other than trauma). Push the patella medially with the outside thumb while stabilizing with the medial thumb (Figure 2–17).

Lateral Displacement of the Patella

Lateral displacement or increased mobility occurs often from injury and postural stress. Push the patella laterally with the medial thumb while using the lateral thumb to control the movement (Figure 2–18).

Care must be taken while testing. If severe lateral mobility is present, either chronic or from injury, the patient will be extremely apprehensive when the patella is pushed laterally (hence the name of this orthopedic test: the apprehension test[1]).

The Q angle, the normal valgus angle, is 10° to 15° in men and 15° to 20° in women.[3] It is the angle formed by the rectus femoris muscle descending medially to the patella and the lateral angle of the descent of the infrapatellar ligament.

The anterior projection of the lateral condyle of the femur provides a fulcrum for the power of the quadriceps femoris muscles while helping retain the patella in the trochlear groove (Figure 2–19).

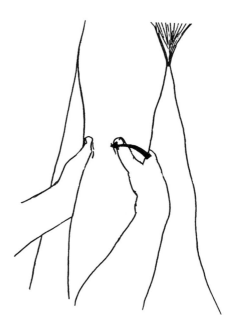

Figure 2–18 Right knee, test for lateral patella stability.

The pressure of pulling laterally by the rectus femoris, vastus intermedialis, and vastus lateralis is offset by the vastus medialis (the largest of the quadriceps). Its oblique fibers are the main medial stabilizers of the patella. These fibers originate lower on the femur than the vastus lateralis and provide stabilization for efficient tracking of the patella in the trochlear groove. Any increase in the Q angle will produce increased stress on the VMO and abnormal tracking of the patella in the trochlear groove.

The stress of the later stages of pregnancy may produce an anteriorly rotated pelvis, a medially rotated femur, a laterally rotated tibia, and an increased Q angle. This may account for

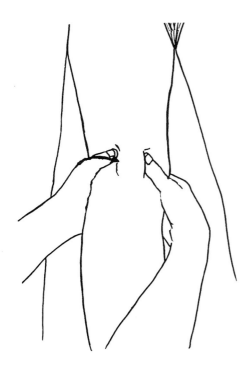

Figure 2–17 Right knee, test for medial patella stability.

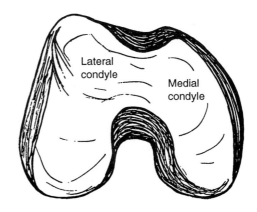

Lateral condyle

Medial condyle

Figure 2–19 Right femur, inferior surface.

some of the chronic knee and back problems in women seen in practice. Any long-term dysfunction of tracking of the patella in the trochlear groove will produce irritation and eventual degeneration.

Lateral displacement of the patella occurs in valgus knee with lateral rotation of the tibia. With lateral rotation of the tibia, the tibial tubercle moves laterally, causing an increased angle of the patellar ligament and placing greater stress on the VMO. Therein lies the reason for atrophy of the VMO in most knee injuries. It has been the author's experience that weakness of the VMO through minor strains and postural fault is one of the most frequent causes of knee symptoms in nontraumatic cases.

If resistance is met while pushing medially, it may be due to increased contraction of the vastus lateralis and tightening of the iliotibial tract. The contraction may be a result of the VMO strain or weakness.

Once the VMO is weak or strained, normal function and general exercises perpetuate the imbalance by overdeveloping the lateral muscles, which are the ones that are more capable of functioning. Palpation of the muscles reveals greater tone and bulk of the vastus lateralis while tone of the VMO and the rest of the vastus medialis is lacking.

In the extended knee, the patella rides above the trochlear groove, resting on the fat pad. The patella is proximal to the projecting lateral condyle, allowing mediolateral palpation for muscle tone or laxity.

Care must be taken when checking for lateral mobility (medial muscle tone). In the apprehension test, when the patella reaches its normal limit and it appears that the examiner is going to push it beyond, the patient will become very apprehensive.

Lateral dislocation of the patella may occur from:

- trauma
- a shallow lateral femur condyle
- a shallow trochlear groove
- chronic increased Q angle
- a combination of any of these

Self-Evaluation

At this point, the author recommends that the student and practitioner alike follow along with self-examinations of the right knee. The intention is to familiarize the reader with the individual structures and to lead to a better understanding of their function.

Hereafter, the self-examinations will appear in text boxes. The clinical examination will remain in regular text. All directions will be on the right knee. Sit in a chair with the right knee extended, and bare the knee joint. Resistance to movement may be provided by the left foot when called for.

Palpation of the Lateral Trochlear Groove

Flex the knee to 100° or more. Flexion moves the patella inferior to the articular surfaces of the femur and exposes the trochlear groove. Palpate along the exposed anterior surface of the lateral condyle before palpating the groove. Palpate along the medial edge of the lateral rim of the groove for areas of pain and edema.

Flex the knee to 100° or more. Flexion moves the patella inferior to the articular surfaces of the femur and exposes the trochlear groove. Palpate along the exposed anterior surface of the lateral condyle before palpating the groove. Injuries that occur by a direct blow to the flexed knee may cause damage to the lower surface of the femur that is not palpable in any other position. Palpate along the medial edge of the lateral rim of the groove for areas of pain and edema (Figure 2–20).

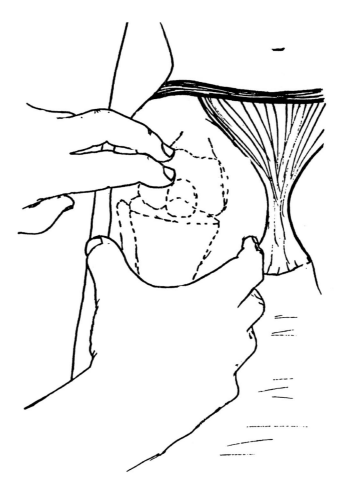

Figure 2–20 Right knee, palpation of the lateral femoral condyle and trochlear groove.

Palpation of the Medial Trochlear Groove

> Palpate the exposed anterior surface of the medial femur condyle before palpating the groove. As with the lateral side, palpate for areas of edema and pain and on the medial side for the possibility of thickening of the plica, which is sometimes associated with chondromalacia.

Palpate the exposed anterior surface of the medial femur condyle before palpating the groove (Figure 2–21). As with the lateral side, palpate for areas of edema and pain and on the medial side for the possibility of thickening of the plica, which is sometimes associated with chondromalacia (see Chapter 6).

Palpation of the Anterior Joint

> Place the knee in 20° of flexion and grasp the tibial condyles, placing the thumbs on the anterior rim of the tibial condyles bilaterally (in the acute case palpation may start at 0°). Palpate the anterior joint structure at several intervals of flexion up to 100°, looking for any tissue abnormality or area of reported pain.

Place the knee in 20° of flexion and grasp the tibial condyles, placing the thumbs on the anterior rim of the tibial condyles bilaterally (in the acute case palpation may start at 0°). Palpate the anterior joint structure at several intervals of flexion up to 100°, looking for any tissue abnormality or area of reported pain (Figure 2–22).

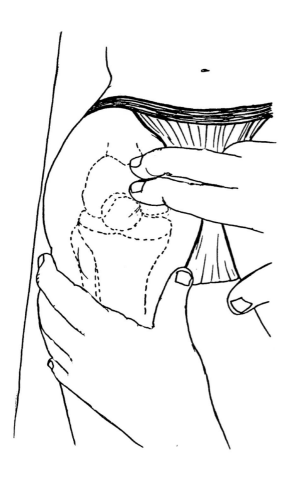

Figure 2–21 Right knee, palpation of the medial femoral condyle and trochlear groove.

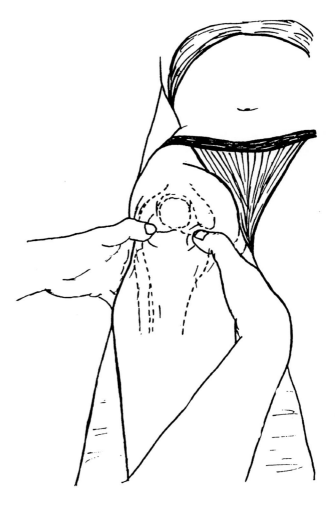

Figure 2–22 Right knee, palpation of the anterior joint.

Laterally Rotated Tibia Fixation

The screw-home movement that allows hyperextension to occur is a result of the medial condyle of the tibia (with its greater articular surface) moving anteriorly from under the femur. This movement occurs from neutral extension to hyperextension and is easily palpated.

Palpation

> Extend the knee to neutral. Place one finger on the anterior surface of the medial condyle of the femur and another on the adjacent tibia condyle. Allow the knee to go into hyperextension. If no fixation exists, the movement of the tibia from under the femur is easily palpated. If a laterally rotated tibia fixation exists, no movement will be palpated.

With the patient's leg resting in neutral extension, place one finger on the anterior surface of the medial condyle of the tibia and another on the medial condyle of the femur. With the footward hand, grasp the ankle and hyperextend the leg (Figures 2–23 and 2–24). The anterior gliding of the medial condyle of the tibia should be felt if no fixation exists. If the medial condyle fails to move anteriorly from under the femoral condyle, it is an indication that rotation occurred in hyperextension but failed to return posteriorly when the knee was returned to neutral extension.

Alternative Method of Palpation for a Laterally Rotated Tibia Fixation

Another method to palpate for a laterally rotated tibia fixation is as follows (Figure 2–25):

1. With the headward hand, grasp the medial condyle of the femur.
2. Apply pressure with the footward hand, using an index finger contact on the medial condyle of the tibia.
3. Simultaneously pull on the femur while pushing posteriorly on the tibia.

Some movement should be palpated unless a fixation is present.

If a laterally rotated tibia fixation exists, the popliteus muscle must be involved in one way or another. As the tibia rotates, the medial condyle moves anteriorly and the lateral condyle acts as a pivot. It is restrained by the ligaments (the anterior cruciate is the strong restraint) and the popliteus muscle. The popliteus muscle is the primary mover of the knee from hyperextension to neutral extension. The knee must reach neutral before the hamstrings become effective. Therefore, the popliteus muscle must be tested after the adjustment.

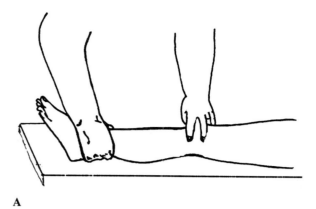

A

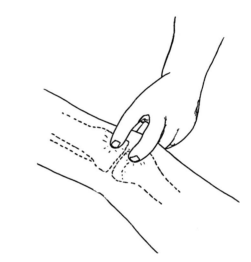

B

Figure 2–23 (**A** and **B**) Contact for palpation of medial condyle motion.

Adductor Tubercle

> Slide the hand down the medial surface of the thigh. The first bone structure encountered is the adductor tubercle. At the beginning of the bone projection is the end of the adductor magnus muscle attachment. Along the projection, slightly inferior and posterior, is the origin of the medial head of the gastrocnemius muscle.

Slide the hand down the medial surface of the thigh. The first bone structure encountered is the adductor tubercle. At the beginning of the bone projection is the end of the adductor magnus muscle attachment. Along the projection, slightly inferior and posterior, is the origin of the medial head of the gastrocnemius muscle (Figure 2–26).

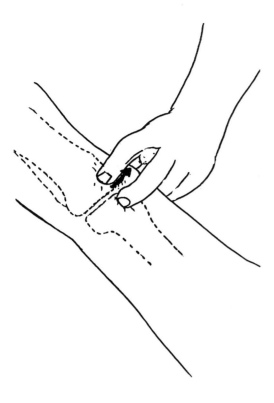

Figure 2–24 Palpation of medial tibial condyle movement.

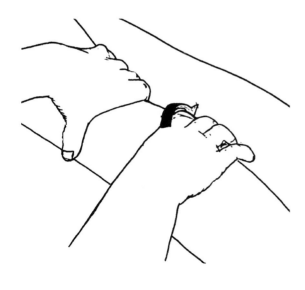

Figure 2–25 Right knee, palpation of lateral rotation fixation.

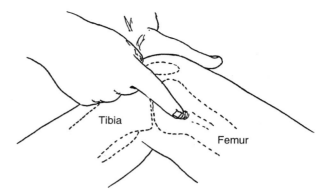

Figure 2–26 Right knee, palpation of the adductor tubercle.

Palpation of the Oblique Fibers of the Vastus Medialis

> Palpate the origin of the VMO using the pads of the fingers of the left hand and starting about two fingers' width above the adductor tubercle.
>
> Palpate *behind* the femur, where the fibers originate They are easily palpated as they pass over the edge of the femur.
>
> On attempting to move the right knee into extension with the foot moving laterally, the fibers may be traced under the sartorius muscle to their insertion on the patella.

Locate the adductor tubercle. The VMO fibers start about two fingers' width above the tubercle on the medial side of the posterior surface of the femur on a level just above the superior border of the patella (Figure 2–27).

The fibers may be palpated deep to the sartorius as they emerge from the posterior femur. To enhance the palpation,

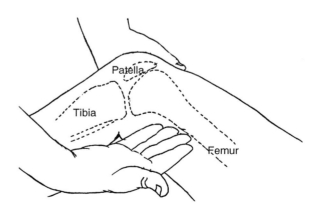

Figure 2–27 Right knee, palpation of the VMO origin.

restrain the foot and ask the patient to attempt movement of the foot slightly laterally while extending the knee.

Medial Collateral Ligament

The origin of the medial collateral ligament (MCL) is just below the adductor tubercle (about one finger's width). The best way to palpate the MCL is by tracing along the medial joint space until the anterior fibers are palpated.

Palpate with the left hand while placing slight valgus stress on the knee with the right hand. By placing stress and then relaxing, the MCL may be easily palpated. By flexing and extending the knee, the fibers may be palpated as they move anteriorly during extension and posteriorly during flexion.

The femoral attachment of the MCL is located below and posterior to the adductor tubercle (Figure 2–28). Locating it may be difficult in the relaxed knee. Palpation is made easier by palpating along the medial joint structures just posterior to the midline. With the patient instructed to relax the leg, move the knee in and out of valgus stress; this will make the middle of the MCL easy to palpate. Once located, the ligament may be traced to its origin on the medial condyle of the femur. Then it may be traced to its insertion on the medial surface of the tibia at the base of the medial condyle (Figures 2–29 and 2–30).

From its origin on the femur, the fibers fan out. Some of the deep fibers attach to the medial meniscus, the capsule, and the tendon of the semimembranosus muscle.

Palpate the attachments and over the entire length for areas of possible rupture. Any interruption in the normal smoothness would indicate a possible rupture and would be painful when palpated.

Several bursae are present under the ligament and should be kept in mind during palpation.

Pes Anserinus

Sartorius

Palpate the anterior medial surface of the medial tibial condyle.

The most anterior attachment on the pes anserinus is the sartorius muscle, lying anterior to the gracilis and the semitendinosus.

Provide resistance with the left foot. Allow passive movement of the knee laterally (this takes away gracilis function). Start to move the right foot toward the opposite knee. The sartorius becomes prominent and may be traced from the insertion all the way to the anterosuperior iliac spine.

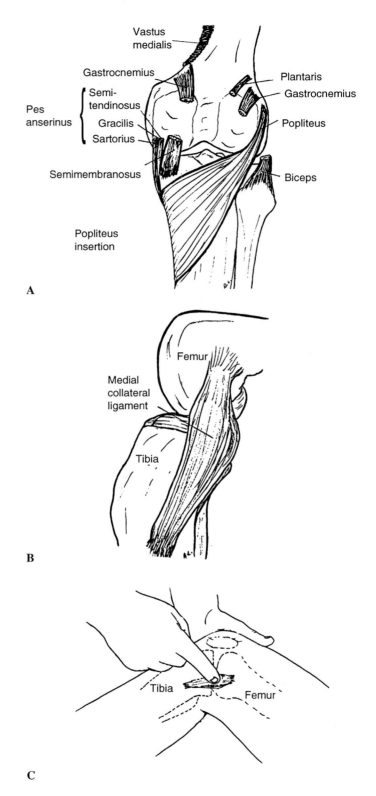

Figure 2–28 (A) Right knee, posterior view showing muscle attachments. **(B)** Right knee, flexed, medial view. **(C)** Right knee, palpation of the MCL.

The sartorius muscle insertion is flat and lies anterior to the gracilis and semitendinosus muscles as they insert into the medial surface of the tibial condyle (Figure 2–31).

To facilitate palpation of the sartorius muscle, restrain the foot from moving, and have the patient gently make the effort to move the foot to the opposite knee. This action makes the sartorius more prominent and easier to identify (Figure 2–32).

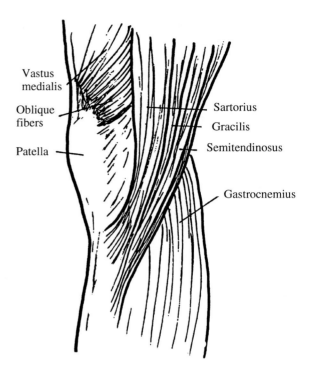

Figure 2–31 Right knee, medial view showing muscle attachments.

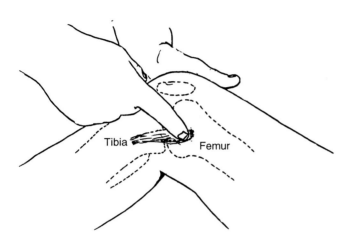

Figure 2–29 Right knee, palpation of the MCL origin.

Gracilis

Cease the sartorius movement. With the knee abducted, provide resistance with the right hand and attempt adduction. The gracilis is the only muscle below the knee joint that adducts. It will become prominent just behind the sartorius insertion.

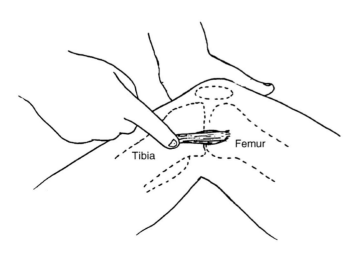

Figure 2–30 Right knee, palpation of the MCL insertion.

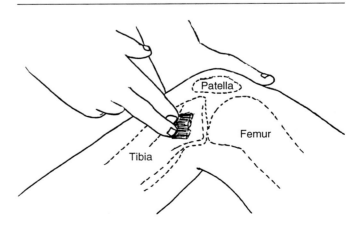

Figure 2–32 Right knee, palpation of the pes anserinus.

Abduct the knee, provide resistance with the palpating hand, and have the patient adduct the knee. The gracilis will become apparent just behind the sartorius insertion. It is the only adductor of the knee below the adductor tubercle.

Semitendinosus

> With the knee flexed to approximately 15°, laterally rotate the right foot. Restrain it from medial movement with your left foot. Without movement of the knee, attempt medial rotation of the foot.
>
> The semitendinosus, lying deep and posterior to the gracilis, will become apparent behind the gracilis. The tendon will stand out because it is a strong medial rotator along with the popliteus.

Flex the knee to approximately 15°. Have the patient laterally rotate the foot. Provide restraint to the foot to prevent medial rotation.

Have the patient attempt medial rotation of the foot. The tendon of the semitendinosus will become apparent behind the gracilis.

Semimembranosus

> Maintain lateral rotation of the right foot without any restraint. Flex the knee, and the semimembranosus becomes apparent as it inserts into the posterior surface of the medial tibial condyle lateral to the semitendinosus (toward the center of the knee joint).

Lying deep to the semitendinosus, the semimembranosus inserts laterally (toward the center of the knee) into the posterior surface of the medial condyle of the tibia (see Figure 2–33).

After locating the semitendinosus, have the patient laterally rotate the foot *without restraint* and hold. Have the patient increase flexion of the knee, and the tendons of the semimembranosus become more prominent.

Palpation of the Popliteus Muscle Insertion

> See Figure 2–33 for the insertion. Use the four fingers of the left hand, and palpate just behind the sharp ridge on the posterior medial tibia just below the medial condyle.
>
> Medially rotate the foot, and the insertion is easily palpated.

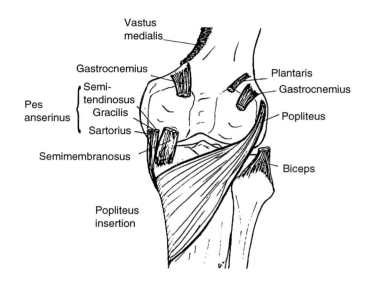

Figure 2–33 Right knee, posterior view showing muscle attachments.

Have the patient laterally rotate the foot and provide restraint. Using four fingers slightly apart (about the size of the insertion), palpate the ridge on the medioposterior tibia just below the condyle.

Have the patient attempt medial rotation several times, and the insertion becomes easily palpated (Figure 2–34).

Moving behind the ridge, the medial portion of the insertion may be palpated on the posterior surface. Palpate the insertion fibers for areas of contraction, areas without muscle tone, and areas of reported pain.

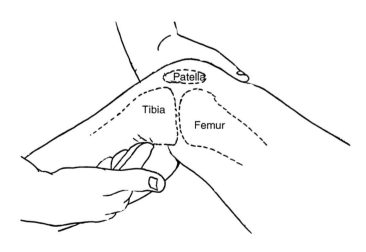

Figure 2–34 Right knee, palpation of the popliteus muscle insertion.

Lateral Structures

Iliotibial Tract

> With the knee flexed, palpate the lateral side of the front joint line. By gently attempting extension, the iliotibial tract may be palpated as the main fibers cross to their insertion on the anterior surface of the lateral tibial condyle. It also attaches to most other structures of the knee.

With the knee still flexed, palpate along the lateral joint line from the front. As palpation proceeds posteriorly, the first structure easily palpated is the iliotibial tract as it crosses the joint (Figure 2–35). Palpation of the tract is helped by retaining the foot in position and asking the patient to attempt extension of the knee.

With the attempt, palpation of the tract is possible to its insertion on the anterior surface of the lateral tibial condyle. Keep in mind that the tract's main insertion is on the condyle; however, it also inserts into other structures. Extend palpation from the lateral thigh, over the lateral femur condyle (an area of possible irritation) to the patella and the fascia of the knee while the patient contracts and relaxes (Figure 2–36).

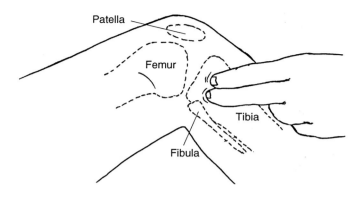

Figure 2–36 Right knee, palpation of the iliotibial tract insertion.

Lateral Collateral Ligament

> With the iliotibial tract located, palpate posteriorly along the joint line, and the next structure crossing the joint is the lateral collateral ligament (LCL).
>
> Move the knee into varus stress with the left hand, and palpation of the LCL becomes easier from the origin to the fibula head (see discussion of the biceps femoris).

With the iliotibial tract located, palpate posteriorly along the joint line, and the next structure crossing the joint is the LCL (Figure 2–37).

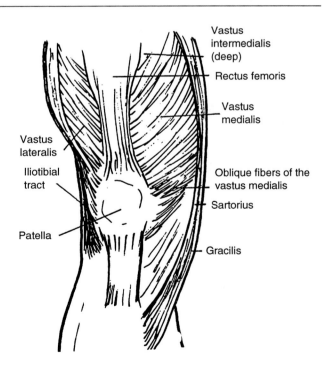

Figure 2–35 Right knee, anterior view.

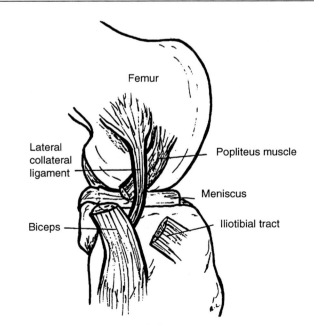

Figure 2–37 Right knee, lateral view.

With the foot on the table, gently apply varus stress to the knee, and the LCL becomes easier to palpate. Palpate to the origin on the lateral condyle of the femur. Palpate all the fibers for tears. Palpate to the insertion on the fibula (Figure 2–38; see discussion of the biceps femoris).

Popliteus Tendon

> Once the LCL is located, find the most posterior fibers at the joint line.
>
> Provide resistance with the left foot, and gently medially rotate the right foot. The popliteus tendon crosses the joint line obliquely just behind the LCL. The tendon comes from under the LCL after originating just inferior and anterior to the LCL origin on the lateral condyle of the femur.

After palpation of the LCL, relax the varus stress, and have the patient gently move the foot into medial rotation against resistance. The origin of the popliteus muscle may be palpated on the lateral condyle of the femur, inferior and slightly anterior (in flexed knee) to the origin of the LCL (Figure 2–39).

Moving across the LCL at the joint line, the tendon of the popliteus muscle may be palpated as it crosses the joint just posterior to the LCL. Alternating contraction and relaxation of the attempted medial rotation of the foot may allow palpation of the popliteus tendon. Lateral femur condyle movement posteriorly (caused by popliteus contraction) may also be palpated.

Palpation along the joint line should include any possible meniscus protrusion and areas of pain and/or edema. It is important to remember that the lateral meniscus is not attached to the LCL but to the popliteus tendon.

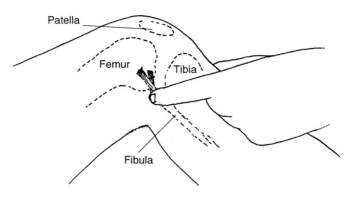

Figure 2–39 Right knee, palpation of the popliteus muscle tendon.

Biceps Femoris

> Flex the knee to 80°, and palpate the biceps tendon as it inserts into the fibula head. It surrounds the LCL insertion, which may now become more apparent by also varus stressing the knee.

After palpation of the lateral joint is completed, provide resistance, and ask the patient to flex the knee more while laterally rotating the foot. The biceps tendon becomes prominent and easily palpated with the effort (Figure 2–40). The biceps inserts into the fibula head surrounding the insertion of the LCL. To help in identifying the insertions, alternately repeat the above contractions with varus stress during each relaxation.

> This is the end of the self-examination portion of this chapter.

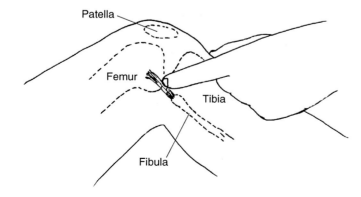

Figure 2–38 Right knee, palpation of the LCL.

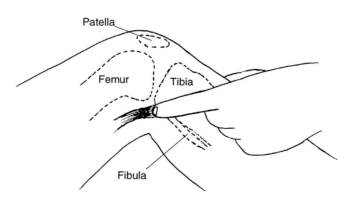

Figure 2–40 Right knee, palpation of the biceps tendon.

Mediolateral Joint Stability

There are many orthopedic tests for the knee, usually listed by the name of the originator of the test. It is the intention of this author to list by name only those that are necessary for communication with other professionals and to discuss the rest by providing a description of the test.

Instability must be ruled out before continuing if:

- trauma is the cause of symptoms
- edema or hemarthrosis is present
- ligamental laxity is suspected

In hyperextension there should be no mediolateral movement. The screw-home movement from neutral to hyperextension tightens the cruciate, capsular, and the collateral ligaments.

With the knee in neutral extension, as it usually is in the supine position, slight mediolateral movement is normal, increasing to 10° to 15° at 30° of flexion.

If the knee will not relax in the supine position and edema is present, all the instability tests must be assumed to have more mobility than tested. The presence of edema, pain, and pain reaction may cloud the results of the tests.[1] All tests should be repeated after the edema has been reduced.

Test for Lateral Joint Stability

Testing for lateral joint stability (or lack of stability) may start in the neutral, relaxed position on the table. Place one hand under the knee, supporting the knee while palpating the lateral joint structure. Grasp the foot and ankle and elevate the leg as a unit, bringing the leg to a position where careful control may be maintained (Figure 2–41).

Slowly allow the knee to drop into hyperextension to the fullest extent tolerated by the patient. A knee with edema may only allow movement to 10° of flexion, and testing would have to begin at that position.

With the knee extended as far as allowed, support the knee with the proximal hand. Provide resistance to the medial knee structure with the fingers, and palpate the lateral joint structure with the thumb while moving the foot and ankle medially. Test first in hyperextension and then in graduated degrees of flexion to approximately 30°.

Excessive joint play in hyperextension would indicate damage to the cruciates, possibly the lateral capsular ligaments, and/or the popliteus muscle. The screw-home movement of hyperextension tightens the cruciates and, if they are intact, will prevent lateral or medial movement even with the collateral ligaments torn. Excessive joint play from neutral extension to flexion would indicate damage to the LCL and/or the popliteus muscle.

Some tests have shown that the popliteus muscle is a strong stabilizer in lateral stability as a result of its tendon attachment on the lateral femur condyle.

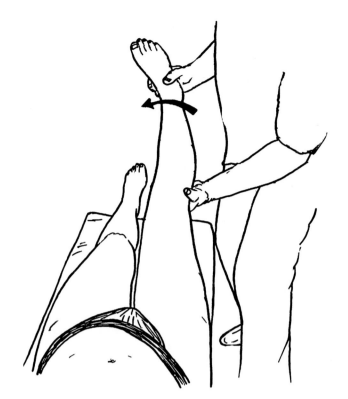

Figure 2–41 Test for lateral joint stability.

Test for Medial Joint Stability

As with the lateral stability test, begin testing for medial stability with the knee in neutral, resting on the table if possible (Figure 2–42).

Elevate the leg to a comfortable position using one hand over the knee and the other hand and wrist under the calf. Control the distal leg with the elbow, holding it against the rib cage. This allows the distal hand to control extension and flexion.

With the proximal hand over the knee (as in Figure 2–42), provide resistance to knee movement with the thumb while palpating the medial joint structures with the middle or index finger. With the knee held in place, abduct the leg to test for instability. As in the test for lateral stability, test in several positions from hyperextension to 30° of flexion.

Injuries may occur with pressure from any direction and with the knee in any degree of flexion, causing a wide variety of tissue damage. Before ligamental damage occurs, there is usually damage to the muscles, tendons, retinaculum, and fasciae. Which structures are injured depends on the degree of flexion and the direction and severity of the trauma. Injuries to tissue other than the ligaments usually produce inflammation and edema that interfere with obtaining clear findings.

Interpreting tests for instability is not without controversy. Most of the controversy concerns which ligaments are in-

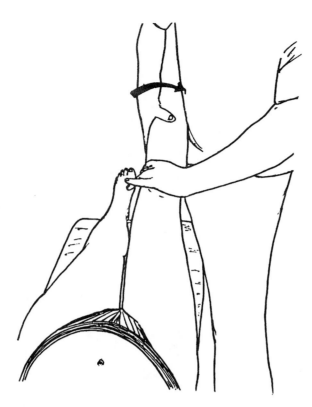

Figure 2–42 Test for medial joint stability.

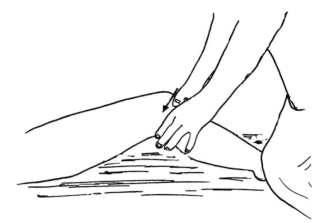

Figure 2–43 Posterior drawer test.

volved. The presence of edema and pain inhibits accurate testing. The author has found a number of clinicians who agree that the initial diagnosis was inaccurate upon subsequent re-examination after swelling had been reduced.

Ellison[4] stated that acute tears of the anterior and posterior cruciates occur commonly without any laxity and that mediolateral testing is a more reliable indicator.

With the two previous paragraphs in mind, sprains may be graded as follows:

1. first degree—no laxity with a few failed fibers
2. second degree—0 to 10 mm increased opening with one-third to two-thirds failed fibers; 5 to 10 mm increased opening, at risk for complete failure and requires immobilization
3. third degree—10 mm increased opening or more with more than two-thirds fiber failure

Posterior Drawer Test

The posterior drawer test is performed with the knee flexed at 90° and the foot in the neutral position (Figure 2–43). Apply posterior pressure to the tibial condyles. A positive posterior drawer test would indicate not only posterior cruciate ligament tearing but also involvement of posterior capsular and arcuate ligaments. Depending on the degree of flexion (or lack

thereof), the popliteus muscle may tear; this should be a consideration in a positive posterior drawer test.

Tearing of the posterior ligament occurs less often than tearing of the anterior ligament. Always compare with the opposite knee.

Anterior Drawer Test

The anterior drawer test is performed with the knee flexed at 90° and the foot stabilized in the neutral position (Figure 2–44). Grasp the tibial condyles and pull anteriorly. Retest with the foot rotated medially, then laterally.

Medial rotation of the tibia tightens the posterolateral capsule; therefore, if the amount of instability found in neutral still exists, it would indicate not only involvement of the anterior cruciate but also posterolateral capsular tearing.

Lateral rotation of the tibia tightens the posteromedial capsule; if the instability found in neutral is still present, it would indicate posteromedial capsular tearing as well.

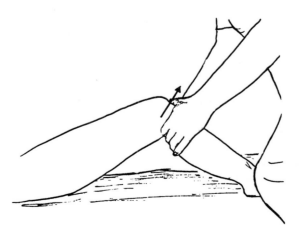

Figure 2–44 Anterior drawer test.

With an intact capsule, medial or lateral rotation would reduce the amount of instability found with the foot in neutral.

When flexing the knee to 90° is not possible, the tests may be modified in several ways.

Lachman's Test

From this position, testing for anterior and posterior ligament stability may be performed.

Place the patient supine or sitting with the distal end of the femur resting on the edge of the padded table end (Figure 2–45). The foot and ankle are placed between the knees of the examiner, and the patient's knee is flexed to 20° to 30°. Grasp the tibial condyles from behind while placing the thumb pads on the femur condyles. Apply mild traction on the leg by leaning back. Pull anteriorly on the tibial condyles while providing resistance on the femur with the thumb pads.

With the distal ends of the femur on the end of the table, apply posterior pressure on the tibial condyles to test for posterior cruciate stability.

Lateral Rotation Instability

With excessive anterior movement of the medial tibia condyle from under the femur (lateral rotation), when the valgus stress test is negative in the extended knee it should be positive with the knee flexed.

To test for lateral rotation instability (Figure 2–46), grasp the medial condyle of the tibia with the footward hand, and flex the knee approximately 5°. With the headward hand, apply posterior pressure on the medial condyle of the femur while simultaneously pulling on the medial condyle of the tibia. Using the thumb, apply posterior pressure on the lateral condyle of the tibia.

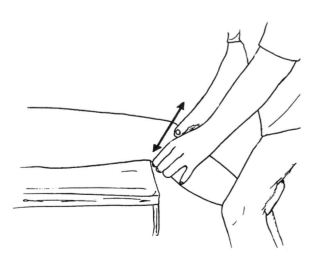

Figure 2–45 Alternative position to perform anterior and posterior drawer tests (Lachman's Test).

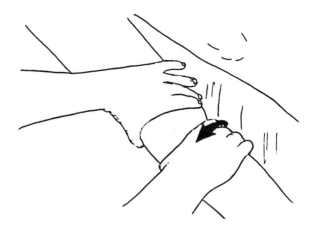

Figure 2–46 Test for lateral rotation instability.

Depending upon the degree of injury, the structures involved are the following:

- popliteus muscle
- medial hamstrings
- VMO
- retinaculum of the medial side of the knee
- MCL (deep fibers)
- capsular ligaments
- anterior cruciate ligament

Again, interpretation of findings is not without controversy. Some consider the anterior cruciate ligament an important proprioceptor that allows the screw-home effect to occur and believe that it is the primary structure involved. Others have found that sectioning the anterior cruciate in a cadaver allowed no greater rotation of the tibia, so that other ligaments of the knee must be suspected. The only accurate method of interpretation, of course, is with the use of magnetic resonance imaging.

Medial Rotation Instability

Excessive anterior movement of the lateral tibia condyle from under the femur (medial rotation instability) may be tested with the examiner standing on the opposite side of the table (Figure 2–47). Grasp the lateral tibia condyle with the footward hand, and flex the knee to approximately 5°. Apply posterior pressure on the lateral femur condyle with the headward hand while pulling anteriorly on the tibial condyle, using the thumb to assist in the rotation movement.

Medial rotation instability is, again, not without controversy. The controversy concerns whether the anterior cruciate ligament is *always* involved. If the varus stress test is negative

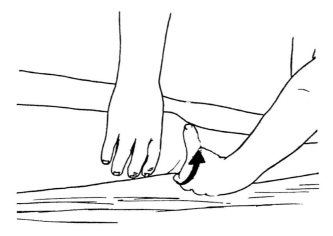

Figure 2–47 Test for medial rotation instability.

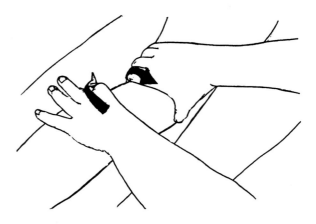

Figure 2–48 Right knee, palpation for medial rotation fixation.

in the hyperextended knee and medial rotation instability exists in flexion, it is reasonable to assume that the anterior cruciate is not involved to any degree.

An excessive anterior displacement of the lateral condyle of the tibia would include damage to several structures depending on the severity of injury:

- iliotibial tract
- biceps femoris (depending on whether the knee was flexed)
- lateral retinaculum
- lateral capsule
- anterior cruciate ligament
- LCL

If no severe rotational instability is found, the examination may continue.

Medial Rotation of the Tibia Fixation

Medial rotation of the tibia fixation occurs less frequently than lateral rotation. One can theorize that the reason is that the Q angle and most of the common stresses produce lateral rather than medial rotational tendencies. The structures of the knee would indicate a difference in occurrence also. The popliteus muscle is a specific muscle to produce medial rotation and to allow lateral rotation. No muscle exists specifically to produce lateral rotation until the knee is flexed far enough for the biceps to take effect.

With the headward hand, grasp the lateral condyle of the femur (Figure 2–48). With the footward hand, use an index contact on the anterior surface of the lateral tibia condyle (use care not to slip to the fibula). Simultaneously pull anteriorly on the femur condyle and posteriorly on the tibia condyle.

Test for Passive Hyperextension

Passive hyperextension is not to be mistaken for genu recurvatum, where the knees (usually both) are congenitally hyperextended.

Grasp both heels and elevate them from the table, keeping them even (Figure 2–49). Observe the knees for the ability to relax into the position. Edema is possible if the knee bounces back to flexion and the screw-home movement does not occur.

If no bouncing back is present, allow the legs to remain suspended. If not painful, ask the patient to try to relax the leg muscles further. Shake the legs gently to check if the patient has relaxed them (Figure 2–50). This provides an opportunity to compare both legs thoroughly and may provide invaluable signs for investigation.

With the muscles consciously relaxed, a comparison of the true bulk of the muscles is possible. Look for obvious muscle contractions, differences in size, the dimpling usually found

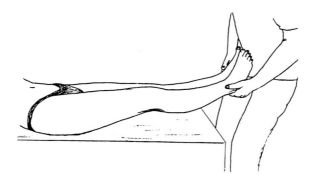

Figure 2–49 Test for passive hyperextension.

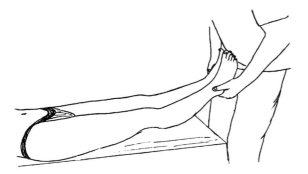

Figure 2–50 Right knee, hyperextended.

medial and superior to the patella (if absent, this is a sign of edema), and atrophy (usually the VMO).

If one knee is hyperextended more than the other, gently press down on each knee, not only feeling for reaction but observing as well (Figure 2–51). If the affected knee is hyperextended, the popliteus muscle must allow it. The seemingly normal knee may be a genu recurvatum that cannot hyperextend because of edema.

Normal hyperextension is 5° to 10°.

Testing the Popliteus Muscle

To test for popliteus muscle strength, flex the knee beyond 100° if conditions allow, place the foot in medial rotation without any inversion, and hold (Figure 2–52A). While the lateral hand supports the heel, with the medial hand take a broad contact on the forefoot, and apply lateral pressure while the patient resists (Figure 2–52B).

Note that the test shown in Figure 2–52 *flexes the knee past 90°*. Testing with the knee at 90° as shown in several texts[5,6] does not take into account the semitendinosus muscle. With the knee at 90° or less, the semitendinosus is a strong medial rotator of the tibia. By flexing past 100° it is removed from efficient functioning.

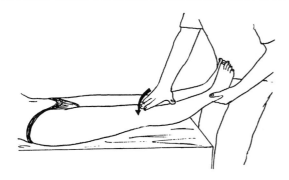

Figure 2–51 Palpation of hyperextended knee.

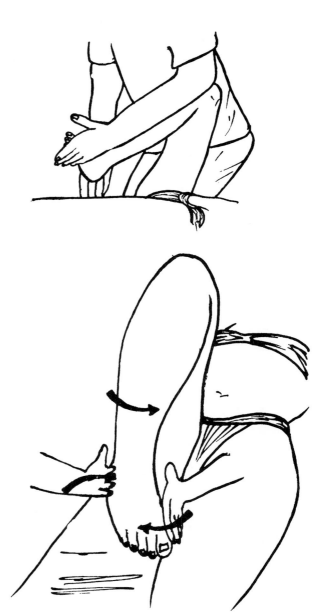

A

B

Figure 2–52 **(A)** Contacts to test the popliteus muscle. **(B)** Popliteus muscle test.

Active Flexion of the Knee

Active flexion of the knee should normally reach 120° with the hip flexed (Figure 2–53).

Passive Flexion of the Knee

Passive flexion (examiner assisted) may reach 160°; the heel may touch the buttocks and should be in line with the ischial tuberosity (Figure 2–54). Patients with large thighs and

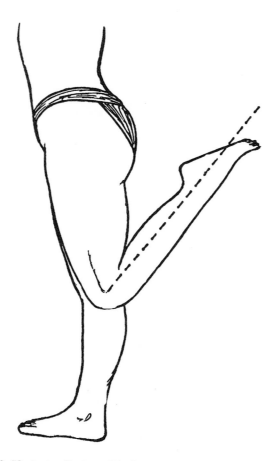

Figure 2–53 Active flexion of the knee to 120°.

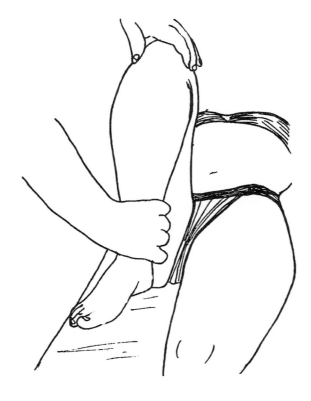

Figure 2–54 Passive flexion of the knee.

calf muscles, such as some bodybuilders, would have restricted flexion.

Passive flexion should allow the same range of motion allowed in squatting.

Rotation of the Lower Leg

Normal rotation of the lower leg, including the tibia, the ankle, and the foot, is normally 30° medially and 40° laterally (Figures 2–55 and 2–56).

Rotation of the Tibia

With the knee at 100°, support the knee with the outside hand while palpating the anterior joint. Grasp the ankle, and rotate medially and then laterally. Normal rotation should be 10° medially and 15° laterally (Figures 2–57 and 2–58).

This eliminates the variance in ankle and foot flexibility.

During the movement, palpate the anterior joint structure for areas of edema, reported pain, and, of course, movement.

With the knee still in 100° of flexion, test for medial and lateral mobility without rotation. Using the same contacts as above and without allowing any rotation to occur, move the ankle medially and then laterally. Ten to fifteen degrees of

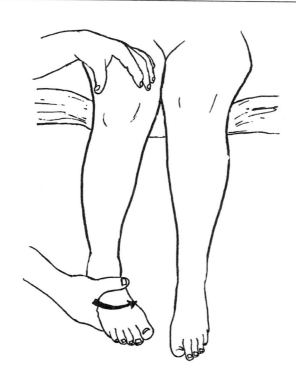

Figure 2–55 Medial rotation to 30°.

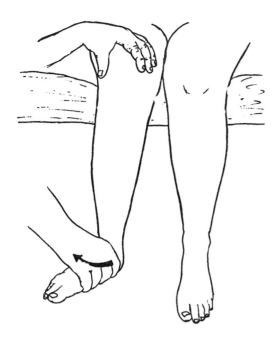

Figure 2–56 Lateral rotation to 40°.

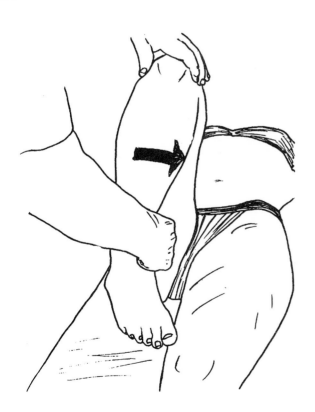

Figure 2–57 Medial tibia rotation.

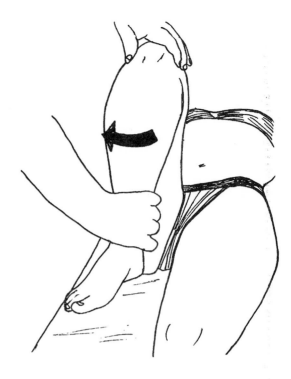

Figure 2–58 Lateral tibia rotation.

mobility in both directions is normal (Figures 2–59 and 2–60). Again, palpate the anterior joint structure for any abnormality.

Palpation of the Medial Meniscus

Return the foot to the table. With the support hand, palpate the medial side of the anterior joint while rotating the foot medially (Figure 2–61).

Medial rotation of the tibia exposes the anterior surface of the medial meniscus and makes palpation of its peripheral attachments easier. Palpate the tibial and femur edge close to the patellar ligament (the area of the transverse ligament).

Palpation of the Lateral Meniscus

Flex the knee to 20°. The joint surface may be palpated along the lateral edge of the tibia and femur for tenderness. Palpation of the lateral meniscus is difficult on the anterior part of the joint structure. By placing varus stress on the joint, however, as in palpation of the LCL, the lateral meniscus may be palpated just posterior to the popliteus tendon.

McMurray's Test for Meniscus Tear

With the knee flexed and the foot near the buttocks, place the support hand in position to apply valgus (medial) pressure, and palpate the joint structure at the same time (Figure 2–62). Grasp the heel and ankle, and laterally rotate the tibia. Apply valgus pressure to the knee while maintaining lateral rotation,

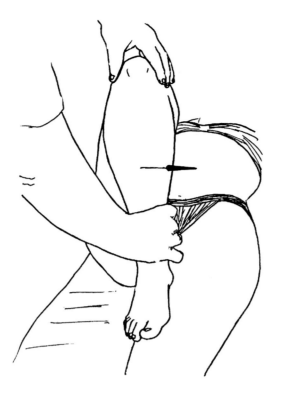

Figure 2–59 Test for medial mobility.

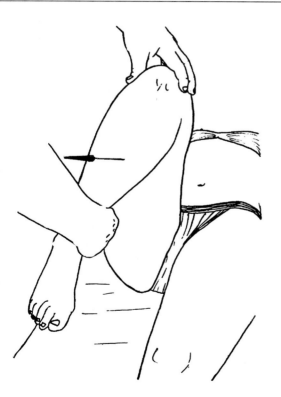

Figure 2–60 Test for lateral mobility.

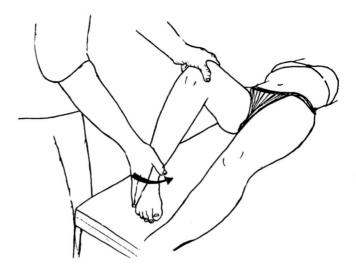

Figure 2–61 Palpation of the medial meniscus.

and slowly extend the knee. The presence of a "click" accompanied by pain indicates the possibility of a medial meniscus tear.

Repeat flexion of the knee, and apply varus pressure while medially rotating the tibia and applying stress to the lateral meniscus.

At the start of McMurray's test, with the knee flexed fully, stress is placed on the posterior section of the respective meniscus. As the knee extends, stress is placed forward to 80°, where the stress is on the middle section. Extension beyond 90° places no stress on the menisci.

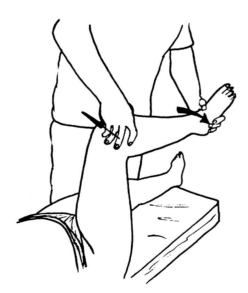

Figure 2–62 McMurray's test.

"Clicking" without pain is not unusual. It may occur while testing for normal rotation and medial to lateral movement of the tibia. Stress, muscle imbalance, and increased pressure from edema interfering with normal movement may produce the "click." In a positive McMurray's test, the "click" is accompanied by pain. Even with pain, however, a positive test only indicates the location of a possible tear.

Extreme weakness of the popliteus and VMO may produce a false-positive McMurray's test.

Testing for Quadriceps Femoris Weakness

Place the knee and hip joints into 90° of flexion. Apply pressure floorward on the ankle while applying pressure on the thigh footward. Floorward pressure on the ankle tests the ability of all four muscles to extend the knee (Figure 2–63). Footward pressure on the thigh tests the rectus femoris muscle, but it also tests the primary hip flexors (to be covered in Chapter 3).

If the ability to extend the knee seems weak (its strength should be substantial) and/or if the movement is painful, repeat only the knee part of the test while supporting the patella medially and superiorly, assisting the VMO (Figure 2–64). If support allows a greater response or a reduction in pain, the VMO function must be addressed.

Neurologic Considerations

Any apparent muscle weakness should lead the examiner to an investigation of possible damage to, instability of, or fixation of the lumbar spine, sacrum, and pelvis.

Cutaneous nerve distributions of the knee area involve L2–5 and S-2. The muscles of the knee are innervated by L-2 to S-2.

Although this text primarily concerns the knee, it cannot be emphasized too much that the body must be treated as a whole. Examination of the spine and pelvis must be included in any

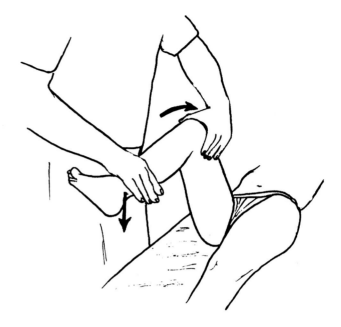

Figure 2–64 Quadriceps femoris test with patellar support.

knee problem. Even a knee injury that conceivably could have occurred when the patient was relaxed and non–weight bearing may involve chronic problems of the spine, pelvis, hip, and foot.

Any trauma involving the lateral aspect of the knee may affect the common peroneal nerve and may include a fibula fracture.

The common peroneal nerve is a branch of the sciatic nerve. It lies between the tendon of the biceps femoris muscle and the lateral head of the gastrocnemius muscle at the level of the fibula head. It winds around the neck of the fibula before dividing into the deep and superficial branches (Figure 2–65).

Trauma directly to the fibula and/or biceps tendon may result in damage to the nerve. Varus-directed traumas with LCL and popliteal muscle tears, allowing excessive separation of the lateral knee, may also result in injury to the common peroneal nerve.

If suspected, look for:

- alterations in cutaneous sensation
- tenderness over the nerve area
- weakness of eversion and dorsiflexion of the foot
- muscle involvement: anterior tibialis, extensor hallucis longus, extensor digitorum longus, and peroneal muscles

To test the patellar reflex, with the patient seated and the lower leg suspended, strike the patellar tendon with a neurologic hammer (Figure 2–66). The reflex should produce movement of the foot forward (knee jerk) and may be graded as normal, increased, decreased, or absent.

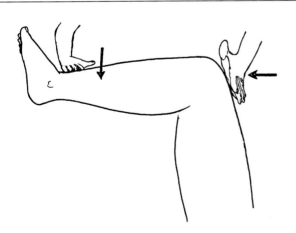

Figure 2–63 Quadriceps femoris test.

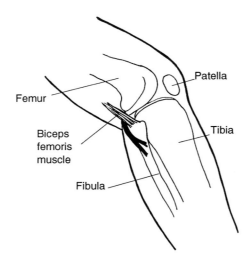

Figure 2–65 Right knee, common peroneal nerve.

The patellar reflex tests the response to stimuli of the quadriceps femoris muscles that includes L2–4, but predominantly L-4 (commonly referred to as the L-4 reflex).

If the patient is supine and/or cannot be tested seated, another method is as follows. With the support hand under the knee, flex the knee approximately 30° to produce minimal tension on the patellar tendon (Figure 2–67). Strike the patellar tendon with the neurologic hammer. If the response is diminished, contact with the support hand allows the examiner to detect even the slightest movement of the knee into extension.

Always compare findings with the opposite knee.

Apley's Compression (or Grinding) Test

Place the patient in the prone position, flex the knee to 90°, and apply pressure on the tibia toward the table (Figure 2–68).

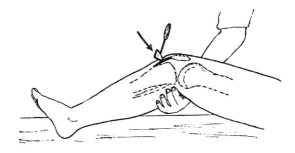

Figure 2–67 Patellar reflex in the supine position.

This applies pressure on both menisci. While applying pressure, rotate the tibia medially and then laterally, applying stress on the ligaments of the knee as well as on the menisci. Pain with pressure alone is a positive sign of the possibility of meniscus damage. Pain upon pressure and rotation may indicate possible ligamental damage as well.

Further Tests To Help Pinpoint Damage

Place the knee into further flexion, move the foot laterally (rotating the femur medially), and apply pressure on the posterior portion of the lateral meniscus (Figure 2–69).

Repeat the procedure, moving progressively into extension to 50°. In extreme knee flexion, pressure is applied to the posterior portion of the lateral meniscus (Figure 2–70). As the knee is moved into lesser degrees of flexion, pressure is placed farther anteriorly to 50°, where the pressure is on the anterior portion of the lateral meniscus.[6]

Repeat as above, moving the foot medially and applying pressure on the posterior portion of the medial meniscus. Again, progressively move the knee to 50°. The compression tests help pinpoint the meniscus damage, if any.

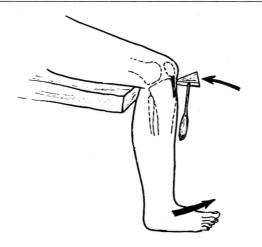

Figure 2–66 Patellar reflex.

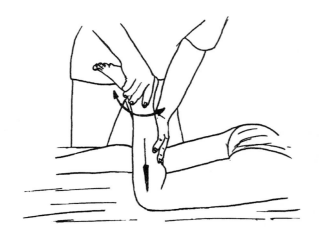

Figure 2–68 Apley's compression test.

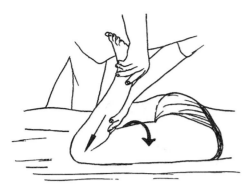

Figure 2–69 Medial rotation of the femur with knee flexion greater than 90°.

Apley's Distraction Test

While securing the femur with the hand or the knee, apply traction on the ankle, removing pressure from the meniscus. Rotation of the ankle applies stress on the capsular and collateral ligaments and helps in differentiating a meniscus from a ligamental tear (Figure 2–71).

If painful with compression but not with distraction, the test would indicate a possible meniscus injury without ligamental damage. If painful with both compression and distraction, the test may indicate that both the meniscus and the ligaments are injured to some degree. If there is no pain with compression but pain on distraction and rotation, the test would indicate possible ligamental damage without meniscus damage.

Fixation

The term *subluxation* has been in the chiropractic profession since the days of DD Palmer. The definition has varied from one school of thought to another.

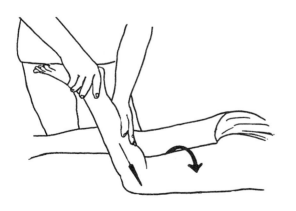

Figure 2–70 Medial rotation of the femur with knee flexion less than 90°.

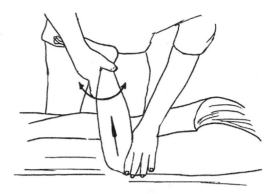

Figure 2–71 Apley's distraction test.

One definition is any articulation that fails to return to its normal resting place. Biron et al[7] refer to a subluxation as simply a slight change in the relative position of a vertebra with its contiguous vertebra. *Dorland's* dictionary defines a subluxation as an incomplete or partial dislocation.

The International Chiropractic Association definition of subluxation is any alteration of the biomechanical and physiologic dynamics of the contiguous spinal structures that can cause neural disturbances. Obviously, this definition does not include any extraspinal structures.

The American Chiropractic Association definition is an aberrant relationship between two adjacent structures that may have functional or pathologic sequelae, causing an alteration in the biomechanical and/or neurophysiologic reflections of these articular structures, their proximal structures, and/or other body systems that may be directly or indirectly affected by them. This definition would include extraspinal structures.

Although not desirous of adding to the controversy, the author, for the purposes of this text, will use the term *fixation*. Fixation may be defined as any articulation that fails to move through its entire normal range of motion.

An articulation may be restricted from movement throughout its normal range of motion by an imbalance of the musculature. The use of static palpation (palpation for position) may determine a malposition of a segment. It will not differentiate between a fixation and a malposition due to muscle imbalance, however.

Passive motion palpation is the application of manual pressure to an articulation without interference from the patient's actions or compensations from weight bearing. If a malposition exists and passive motion palpation produces movement through the normal range of motion, no fixation exists. The malposition is produced by muscle imbalance and should be investigated accordingly.

If the articulation fails to move through its entire normal range of motion on passive motion palpation, a true fixation exists and may be graded as follows:

- severe—0° of movement in the direction tested

- moderate—minimal movement
- mild—moves yet fails to go through the *entire* range of motion

The examiner should keep in mind that if a fixation exists it may have occurred as a result of a muscle imbalance. The examiner should also keep in mind that the restriction of motion may have caused a muscle reaction.

Medial Rotation of the Tibia Fixation

Medial rotation of the tibia fixation occurs less frequently than lateral rotation. One can theorize that the reason is that the Q angle and most of the common stresses produce lateral rather than medial rotational tendencies. The structures of the knee would indicate a difference in occurrence also. The popliteus muscle produces medial rotation and allows lateral rotation; however, no muscle exists specifically to produce lateral rotation (the biceps femoris and iliotibial tract do not function as rotators until flexion).

With the headward hand, grasp the lateral condyle of the femur (Figure 2–72). With the footward hand, use an index contact on the anterior surface of the lateral tibia condyle (take care not to slip to the fibula). Simultaneously pull anteriorly on the femur condyle and posteriorly on the tibia condyle.

Laterally Rotated Tibia Fixation

The screw-home movement that allows hyperextension to occur is a result of the medial condyle of the tibia (with its greater articular surface) moving anteriorly from under the femur. This movement occurs from neutral extension to hyperextension and is easily palpated.

Palpation. With the patient's leg resting in neutral extension, place one finger on the anterior surface of the medial condyle of the tibia and another on the medial condyle of the femur. With the footward hand, grasp the ankle and hyperextend the leg (Figures 2–73 and 2–74). The anterior gliding of

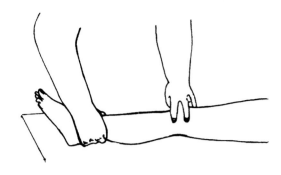

A

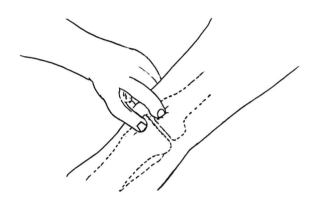

B

Figure 2–73 (A and **B)** Contact for palpation of medial condyle motion.

the medial condyle of the tibia should exist. If the medial condyle fails to move anteriorly from under the femoral condyle, it is an indication that rotation occurred in hyperextension, but failed to return posteriorly when the knee was returned to neutral extension.

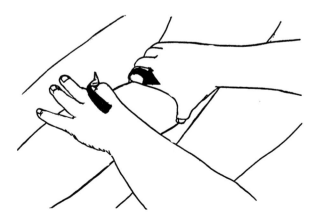

Figure 2–72 Right knee, palpation for medial rotation fixation.

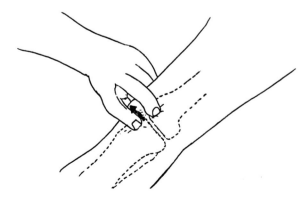

Figure 2–74 Palpation of medial tibial condyle movement.

Alternate Method of Palpation for a Laterally Rotated Tibia Fixation. Another method to palpate for a laterally rotated tibia fixation is as follows (Figure 2–75).

1. With the headward hand, grasp the medial condyle of the femur.
2. Apply pressure with the footward hand, using an index finger contact on the medial condyle of the tibia.
3. Simultaneously pull on the femur while pushing posteriorly on the tibia.

Some movement should be palpated unless a fixation is present.

If a laterally rotated tibia fixation exists, the popliteus muscle must be involved in one way or another. As the tibia rotates, the medial condyle moves anteriorly and the lateral condyle acts as a pivot. It is restrained by the ligaments (the anterior cruciate is the strong restraint) and the popliteus muscle. The popliteus muscle is the primary mover of the knee from hyperextension to neutral extension. The knee must reach neutral before the hamstrings become effective. Therefore, the popliteus muscle must be tested after the adjustment.

Mediolateral Fixations

Seldom does the lateral fixation occur that is not associated with a lateral rotation of the tibia and cannot usually be corrected with a laterally rotated tibia adjustment.

While supporting the knee into slight flexion, apply medial pressure on the lateral condyle of the tibia (make sure not to contact the fibula head) and lateral pressure on the medial condyle of the femur (Figure 2–76). In the slightly flexed knee, some slight "give" should be felt normally.

Medial fixations are palpated in a similar manner (Figure 2–77).

Fibula Fixations

Normal movements of the fibula head are as follows:

- superior

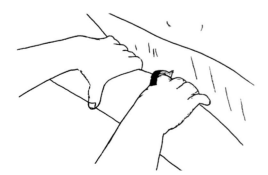

Figure 2–75 Right knee, palpation for lateral rotation fixation.

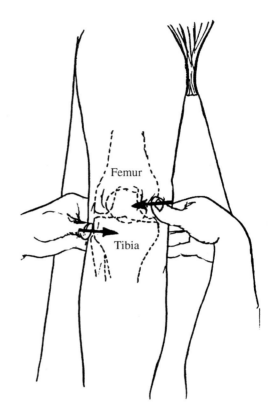

Figure 2–76 Right knee, palpation for lateral fixation of the tibia.

- superoposterior
- anteroinferior
- inferior

Motion Palpation. With the knee extended, palpate the fibula head while dorsiflexing the ankle (Figure 2–78). Failure of the fibula head to move indicates that it is fixed but does not determine whether the fixation is superior or inferior. A determination must be made by:

- comparison with the opposite side for height
- palpation for spasm of the muscles that would retain the fibula distally
- palpation of the biceps femoris muscle insertion on the fibula head for pain and the tendon for a possible hypertonic condition that may be retaining the fibula proximally
- application of pressure inferiorly and then superiorly to determine which direction is restricted

The following is the most accurate method. It allows the examiner to determine not only the superoinferior movement but also the more subtle anteroposterior components. At the same time the function (or lack of function) of the muscles involved can be detected.

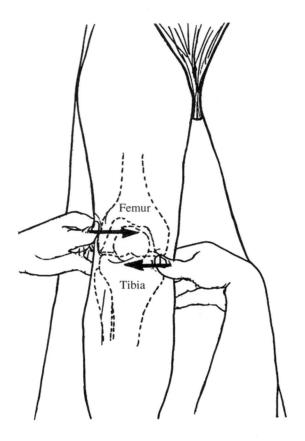

Figure 2–77 Right knee, palpation for medial tibia fixation.

With the knee flexed in the supine position, palpate the fibula head, and begin with the knee only slightly flexed. Dorsiflex the ankle to palpate the normal superior glide of the fibula head during dorsiflexion.

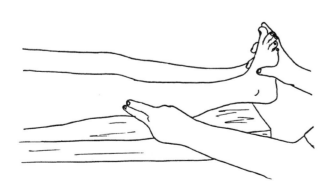

Figure 2–78 Palpation of the fibula head while dorsiflexing the ankle.

Have the patient dorsiflex the ankle while providing resistance. During resisted dorsiflexion of the ankle, the fibula is drawn inferiorly and anteriorly by the extensor digitorum longus, peroneus brevis, peroneus tertius, and extensor hallucis longus muscles.

Have the patient dorsiflex the ankle and flex the knee. If attempted flexion of the knee is introduced with dorsiflexion of the ankle, the stronger biceps femoris muscle will shift the fibula head superiorly with the leg extended.

Repeat the procedure as several degrees of flexion are introduced. As flexion is introduced, the biceps pulls more posteriorly rather than superiorly, overpowering the other muscles, which have only slight anterior influence compared with the biceps.

With the ankle in dorsiflexion, have the patient attempt plantar flexion against resistance. During plantar flexion the fibula is drawn inferiorly and posteriorly by action of the flexor hallucis longus, soleus, and posterior tibialis muscles.

During each of the movements, the examiner has an opportunity to palpate not only the possible fixation but muscle dysfunction as well. Muscle dysfunction may lead to problems of the foot and ankle that may be contributing to or be caused by the knee problem.

Palpation of the Fibula Head while Sitting. In the seated position, the ankle may be dorsiflexed and plantar flexed as necessary (Figure 2–79).

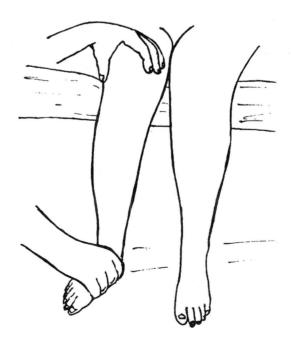

Figure 2–79 Palpation of the fibula head in sitting position.

Exhibit 2-1 Knee Examination Form

Knee Examination

Name: _____   Age: _____   M   F   Date: _____

Occupation: _____   Ambulatory?   Y   N   With pain?   Y   N

Gradual onset?   Y   N   If yes, starting _____   Sudden onset?   Y   N   When? _____

If an injury, describe _____

_____

Key: ✗ Point of pain   ◯ Edema   〰〰 Hypertonic   ⊢——⊣ Stretch   ↗ Direction
       ✗ Pain on performance   ⊓ No tone

Prone sleeper?   Y   N   If yes,   L   R

Rise to stand on both legs _____

Rise to stand   Lt _____   Rt _____   Squat _____

Patella   Lat _____   Alta _____

Patella pain?   Y   N   _____ degree of flexion

Tibial tuberosity _____   Patella ligament _____

Instability   Med _____   Lat _____

Rotator instability   Med _____   Lat _____

Drawer   Ant _____   Post _____

Fixations: Rotated tibia   Lat _____   Med _____

        Tibia   Lat _____   Med _____

Range of   Hyperextension (–10) _____   Standing active (120) _____   Active with hip (140) _____   Passive (160) _____

Motion   Rotation with foot   Lateral (40) _____   Medial (30) _____   Tibia rotation lateral (15) _____   Medial (10) _____

Medial	**Lateral**	**Anterior**	**Tests**
Anterior joint _____	Anterior joint _____	QL hyper _____	McMurray's _____, _____ degrees
Anterior ligament _____	Iliotibial tract _____	QL strain _____	QF test _____
Adductor tuberosity _____	LCL origin _____	Patella compress _____	QF test with support _____
VMO origin _____	LCL _____	Degree of flex _____	QF-thoracic fix _____
MCL origin _____	Popliteus tendon _____	Trochlear groove _____	Popliteus test _____
MCL _____	Lateral meniscus _____	Lateral _____ Medial _____	Popliteus with T4-5 _____
MCL insert _____	Biceps tendon _____	Distal femur Rt _____ Lt _____	Sartorius test _____
Medial meniscus _____	Fibula head _____		Gracilis test _____
Pes anserinus _____	Fibula fixation Sup _____		Hamstrings Lateral _____
Sartorius _____	Sup-Post _____ Inf. _____		Medial _____
Gracilis _____	Inf-ant. _____		Apley comp. Lateral _____
Semitendinosus _____			Medial _____
Semimembranosus _____			Apley distract _____
Popliteus _____			Knee jerk _____
			Comm. peroneal N. _____

Diagnosis: _____

Recommended treatment: Tape-QF _____   Popl _____   MCL _____ Sart-Grac _____   Pes anserinus _____   LCL _____   Biceps _____

   Exercises: VMO _____   Popl _____   Sart-Grac _____   Biceps _____   Med Ham _____   LLS _____

   Ice _____   Moist heat _____   US _____

Prognosis: _____   Next visit: _____

Comments: _____

_____   Dr. _____

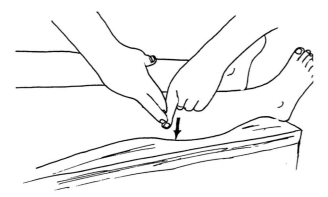

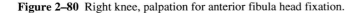

Figure 2–80 Right knee, palpation for anterior fibula head fixation.

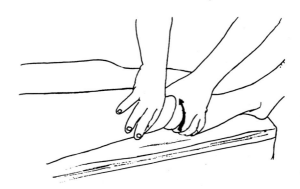

Figure 2–81 Right knee, palpation for posterior fibula head fixation.

Palpation for an Anterior Fixation. Another method of palpating for a lack of posterior movement (anterior fixation) is to use the pad of a finger on the anterior fibula head to make contact and provide a surface for applying pressure. With the other hand, apply pressure posteriorly to palpate for fixation (Figure 2–80).

Palpation for a Posterior Fixation. To test for anterior glide (posterior fixation), support the tibial condyles with one hand. Grasp the fibula head, and pull anterolaterally against resistance (Figure 2–81).

EXAMINATION FORM

Exhibit 2-1 is an examination form, which is necessary for recording the findings. Without a form, writing down the findings often takes longer than the examination. This form follows the procedures as outlined and in the order described in this chapter. By using symbols as indicated in the key (other symbols may be used if desired), the findings may be marked easily during the examination.

REFERENCES

1. Hoppenfeld S. *Physical Examination of the Spine and Extremities.* New York: Appleton-Century-Crofts; 1976.
2. Turek SL. *Orthopaedics, Principles and Their Application.* Philadelphia: Lippincott; 1967.
3. Kuland DN. *The Injured Athlete*, 2nd ed. Philadelphia: Lippincott; 1988.
4. Ellison AE. *Athletic Training and Sports Medicine.* Chicago: American Academy of Orthopedic Surgeons; 1985.
5. Hammer WI. *Functional Soft Tissue Examination and Treatment.* Gaithersburg, Md: Aspen; 1991.
6. Davies GJ, Larson R. Examining the knee. *Physician Sportsmed.* 1978;4.
7. Biron WH, Wells BF, Houser RH. *Chiropractic Principles and Technic.* Chicago: National Chiropractic College; 1939.

Muscle testing is essential in the examination of all musculoskeletal problems. A muscle imbalance becomes an important objective finding when it verifies subjective complaints, history, observations of functional tests, and findings on palpation. Muscle weakness, when found to be a causative factor, becomes important when one is implementing the correct treatment program.

Testing of an individual muscle is difficult. The attempt to isolate a primary muscle also includes the stabilizers and the secondary support muscles.

Muscle testing is the continuation of an active movement by the patient, with the examiner using his or her skill to provide resistance. Resistance should be from a position and in a direction to elicit the greatest response by the *primary* muscle. The skilled examiner will observe the patient's effort and the body's reaction during the attempt.

GRADING

Grading of muscle strength is based on the Lovett system from 1932 as reported by Kendall[1]:

0—no contraction
1—muscle contraction without movement
2—movement produced with elimination of gravity
3—movement against gravity
4—movement against gravity as well as against resistance
5—movement that will overcome a greater amount of resistance

Movement of a joint requires a prime mover or movers, secondary movers, stabilizers of the joint, and secondary support muscles (muscles that stabilize the bone structure from which the movers originate).

A lack of normal strength in muscles other than the prime mover may give the following findings:

- Testing of the primary may seem normal yet is accompanied by shifting of body position to give the secondary muscles greater advantage.
- Testing of the primary may seem normal yet is accompanied by abnormal muscle reaction by the patient, such as shaking of the limb during the test or, if the lower limb is being tested, grasping of the table to assist in the resistance.
- The prime mover may test weak when a weakness of a secondary muscle does not secure the origin, thus interfering with the normal response. For example, testing of the hip flexors (psoas or iliacus) in the presence of a weakness of the iliocostalis lumborum muscle on the opposite side will result in what tests as weak hip flexors. It will also be accompanied by abnormal abdominal movement during the test.

Other factors involved in muscle testing that must be considered are as follows. The patient must understand the test being made. Place the patient in a position in which the muscle being tested has its greatest advantage, and have the patient hold the position. Using an open hand, indicate the direction in which pressure is to be applied. Do not grasp the limb. Grasping makes it difficult for the patient to understand the correct direction. Apply slight pressure, and instruct the patient to resist the movement unless it is painful to do so. Do not "pounce" on it. Gradually increase pressure to maximum so that the patient has the opportunity to react. The object of the test is not to see whether the muscle may be overpowered but to determine whether the response corresponds with normal expectations from a patient of the same size, age, and build. Both extremities should be tested and the affected limb compared with the opposite one.

A judgment must be made as to whether the patient is making the effort called for. This of course is difficult to judge without experience. It is helpful to test other muscles away from the area of complaint first to experience the patient's effort and strength for comparison.

Comparing muscle strength from one side to the other is relatively easy in the normal person. When testing an unusually strong person, such as a bodybuilder, a greater amount of pressure must be applied. If positioned properly and if pressure is applied in the correct direction, any muscle or group of muscles may be overcome, even by a small examiner. Comparison with the opposite side with observations for imbalance in the erect posture and comparisons of muscle tone are essential to obtaining the correct diagnosis. Muscle *balance*, not strength, is the key to comfort.

Muscle tests must not be prejudged by the examiner. Just because a knee is hyperextended in the erect posture, do not assume that the popliteus muscle is weak. It may be hyperextended, but the examiner must keep an open mind to be free to test and observe objectively.

Pain during any part of the test negates the test. It is important to observe the patient closely for reaction and to question the patient. Some patients will not report pain unless asked and will simply make the effort because they were asked to. If pain is present, it is important to know what part of the test became painful and the exact location of the pain. If the muscle tests strong yet pain is present, locating the pain may be helpful in identifying a small muscle tear, tendinitis, or bursitis. Pain away from the primary joint being tested might indicate a problem in the support structure.

Recruitment of other muscles may be necessary to perform the test. Most movements of the body are carried out with ease and smoothly and, against resistance, with strength. In the presence of pain, joint dysfunction, or muscle weakness the body cannot function efficiently and will be forced to use alternative methods to achieve movement when commanded to do so. Normal movement is now replaced with whatever is necessary to carry out the command. Shifting of the body or unusual movements of other musculature may occur to provide greater leverage to other muscles recruited for the function (for want of a better term, the author refers to the unusual movements as cheating). The normally smooth movement may now be supplanted by abnormal direction or hesitation during movement. Subtle alterations of direction by the pa-

tient must be detected and corrected by the examiner. Only with a knowledge of what normal movement is can an examiner detect abnormal movement.

To aid in determining whether a secondary muscle is at fault, give manual assistance to the muscle, or do the job of stabilizing the structure while retesting the primary muscle. If in doubt, retest. A single effort is representative of the patient's ability to perform only once and does not represent the ability to perform the action repeatedly. In injury cases where muscle weaknesses are detected, the author has found that the muscle test should be performed four times consecutively. The fourth test should be normal before the patient is released to return to normal work. If the examiner depends upon only one test, the patient may return to work, perform normally for a short time, and then exacerbate the condition with repeated activity.

Several instruments have been developed in the attempt to test muscles, record findings, and place a numeric grade on muscle tests. Although interesting, each apparatus tested by the author is still dependent upon the skill of the operator, and each of the factors mentioned above must still be considered.

One method is often helpful when a muscle is weaker than expected. After testing, goad (deep moving pressure applied without moving the contact over the skin) the origin and insertion of the muscle and retest. If a muscle has had a mild stretch and is just not functioning up to par, the muscle may respond to goading, and that may be all that is necessary. If a muscle is truly weak, goading the origin and insertion may cause a response. Although the response is only temporary, it may aid in diagnosing the problem.

A muscle that does not respond up to expectations:

- may be mildly stretched as a result of loss of habit pattern and use during activities (eg, abdominal muscles postpartum; stretching during pregnancy alters the habit pattern of use and, if not restored, may result in chronic weakness)

- may be mildly stretched sufficiently to inhibit normal function (eg, stretching of the popliteus muscle while sitting with heels resting on a footstool)

- may simply be weak from lack of use and test weaker than its opposite or its antagonistic muscle

- may be inhibited as a result of fixations (eg, dorsiflexion of the ankle and an anterior atlas fixation in its relationship to the occiput; gluteus maximus abnormality and L-5 fixation)

- may be affected by organic problems (see Appendix A)

- may test weak when it is actually hypertonic (often a hypertonic psoas will test weak, as demonstrated by a positive Thomas test)

- may test weak if there is a loss of fulcrum (as in the quadriceps with a lateral patella)

- may have undergone trauma causing various degrees of damage and muscle reaction

TRAUMA

Trauma may be characterized as follows:
- minimal stretching without fiber damage, inhibiting normal muscle function (may require nothing more than a reminder to return to work with mild exercise)
- trauma sufficient to cause a reaction yet with no fiber damage (eg, a "knuckle" into the deltoid may only require rest, mild stretching, and/or little therapy to return to normal)
- minimal strain—few fibers torn (may respond to 80% of normal; may have minimal pain during the test; no lesion may be palpated in the muscle)
- moderate strain—tear sufficient to allow location by palpation (test produces pain and no response)
- Severe—large depression in the muscle (a large segment is torn and may need surgical repair)

Tears may occur within the bulk of the muscle or at the junction of the muscle and tendon. The tendon can tear, the muscle can tear away from its bone insertion, the tendon can tear away from its bone insertion, or a periosteal separation can occur at the origin or insertion.

SPECIFIC MUSCLE TESTS

Although the examiner must keep in mind the many things that may influence a test, the ability to test the muscle and to determine whether it is normal or not is important. If a muscle fails to respond normally, the examiner has many options to follow up to investigate why and to assist in a proper diagnosis and treatment program.

Quadriceps Femoris

The origins of the three vastus muscles are on the femur. The origin of the rectus femoris is on the anteroinferior iliac spine and the groove just above the rim of the acetabulum (Figure 3–1). To test all four muscles at the same time, it is necessary to test the hip flexors as well.

With the hip and knee at 90°, place one open hand above the knee and one on the ankle (Figure 3–2). Begin by testing the hip flexors with pressure inferior on the knee and minimal pressure on the ankle. If the hip flexor part of the test seems weak, stop the test. If the primary hip flexors (psoas and iliacus) are weak, a rectus femoris weakness is difficult to differentiate. If the primary hip flexors are normal (tested as such) and the first part of the test is weak, it would indicate a weak rectus femoris. Usually with normal hip flexors and a weak rectus, pelvic and/or abdominal movement will occur during the test.

To test the vastus muscles (and, to some degree, the rectus), stabilize the knee with the support hand, and apply pressure on

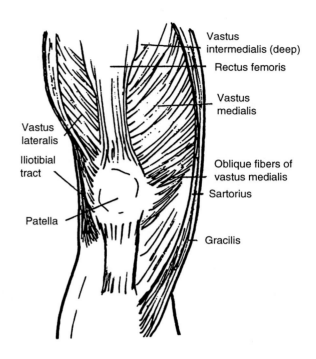

Figure 3–1 Right knee, anterior view.

the ankle only. If the hip flexors seem adequate, apply pressure to extend the hip, and flex the knee at the same time.

To place emphasis on the vastus lateralis (VL), rotate the foot medially and apply pressure into flexion and slightly medially.

To place emphasis on the vastus medialis, laterally rotate the foot, and apply pressure into flexion and slightly laterally.

If the quadriceps test is weak, the first suspect must be the oblique fibers of the vastus medialis muscle (VMO). To test for VMO weakness, retest the quadriceps while supporting the patella medially and slightly proximally (Figure 3–3). Hook the thumb of the support hand around the patella and the

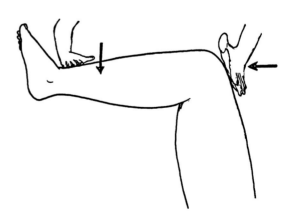

Figure 3–2 Quadriceps femoris test.

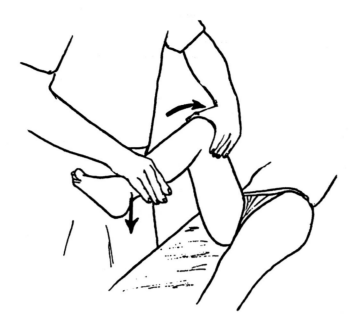

Figure 3–3 Quadriceps femoris test with support.

fingers toward the origin of the VMO (the origin may be painful). Duplicate the action of the VMO while repeating the test. A minimal response may indicate that other problems are more prominent.

A good response would indicate that the VMO is a major factor in producing the symptoms. If the response is positive, repeat the test without support and again with support. This not only will reinforce the diagnosis but also will demonstrate to the patient that one source of the problem has been found.

The author has found the VMO to be a major factor not only in diagnosing the problem but also in establishing a treatment program (see Chapter 6).

Injury to the VMO occurs in many sports, especially in the football clipping injury, where the knee is struck from the side and rear. It occurs in any injury where undue stress is placed on the knee while flexed with the foot laterally rotated (common in skiing injuries). Postural faults with valgus strain taxing normal VMO function may produce microtrauma, stretching, weakness, and susceptibility to harm, even in minor injuries.

Weakness also occurs in the VL, interfering with normal quadriceps function, but this is relatively rare. Seldom does postural distortion place undue stress on the VL. To strain the VL requires a blow the opposite of the clipping injury. An example is the patient in full stride with the one leg forward who is struck on the medial side of the knee by a running dog. If weakness of the VL is suspected, test the VL while supporting the patella and the VL opposite the VMO support.

Testing may be performed in all degrees of flexion if the following is kept in mind:

- Testing the quadriceps femoris forces the patella into the trochlear groove, and the presence of edema or other problems may produce pain. If so, the test should be discontinued.
- Upon testing, some stress is placed on the meniscus. The greater the degree of flexion, the more posterior the pressure. Without pain at 90° and with pain at greater flexion, a posterior meniscus lesion is a possibility.
- There is no constant activity of the muscles during extension, with each muscle performing differently at different degrees of extension.
- Some investigators suggest that the VMO is only effective in the last 20° to 30° of extension. On the basis of the testing method above and other clinical tests, the author has clinically proven otherwise. The VMO is a strong stabilizer at 90° of flexion and is an important factor in returning from a squat at full flexion, especially in the individual with a shallow lateral femoral condyle.

The nerve supply to the quadriceps is the femoral nerve, L2–4. If the weakness is suspected as a result of a fixation, the author has found that correcting fixations of T10–12 and L-1 rather than fixations of L2–4 will affect quadriceps function. One theory is that a fixation affects the muscles and circulation of the articulations of the vertebrae above and below.

A weakness of the quadriceps may be a sign of dysfunction of the small intestines (especially the duodenum; see Appendix A). If so, the area to adjust would be the lower six thoracics. The patient should be questioned about intestinal or digestive distress.

Gracilis and Sartorius

Both these muscles cross the hip and knee joints and have a common insertion in the pes anserinus on the tibia (Figure 3–4). Testing either muscle alone is difficult.

Gracilis

The broad origin of the gracilis on the lower pubis and its descent to the tibia make it the most superficial of the adductor muscles. Its insertion into the pes anserinus allows it to participate in adduction of the hip. It is not a strong adductor, yet it assists by adducting the tibia. With the knee extended, the gracilis provides medial stabilization of the knee. It assists the hamstring muscles in knee flexion after flexion is initiated by the popliteus and hamstrings. Finally, it assists the hamstring muscles in medial rotation of the tibia. Its nerve supply is the femoral nerve (L-2 and L-3).

Sartorius

The sartorius originates from the anterosuperior iliac spine. As a narrow band, it crosses the anterior thigh and over the

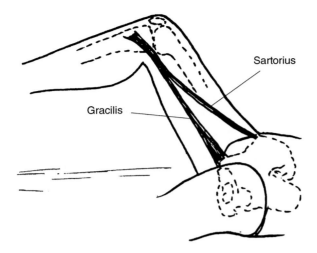

Figure 3–4 Gracilis and sartorius muscles.

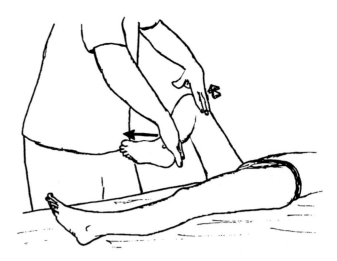

Figure 3–5 Testing the sartorius and gracilis muscles.

vastus medialis muscle on its way to the pes anserinus insertion on the tibia. The sartorius assists in flexion of the hip and knee, abduction of the thigh, and lateral rotation of the thigh. With the knee extended, it assists in stabilization of the knee.[2-4]

The sartorius is referred to as the tailor's muscle because of its function of moving the extended leg to place the ankle on the opposite knee. The sartorius nerve supply is the femoral nerve (L-2 and L-3).

Testing must include both muscles. With the patient in the supine position, place the heel above the opposite knee and abduct approximately 40°. Have the patient hold the position. Place an open hand over the medial aspect of the knee, signaling to the patient that an abduction and slight extension pressure will be made. Place an open hand on the heel and ankle, signaling that pressure to extend the leg with slight abduction from the midline will be made (Figure 3–5).

With the patient resisting, apply pressure with both hands simultaneously. The hand on the knee will feel the response from the gracilis more than the sartorius. The hand on the ankle will feel more of the response from the sartorius.

While testing, it is important to remember that both muscles attach on the pelvis, requiring different secondary support muscles. Compare with the normal knee for abnormal pelvic movements during the test, whether or not the muscles tested weak. Weakness of the gracilis may produce an attempt by the body to extend the hip, enabling the adductors to assist in the test. Weakness of the sartorius may be accompanied by a posterior shifting of the ilium during the test.

A weakened sartorius must be considered in persistent posterior rotation fixations of the ilium. A persistent sartorius weakness may be a sign of adrenal problems (see Appendix A). If adrenal problems are suspected, the specific area to adjust is T-9.

Popliteus

The popliteus originates from the lateral condyle of the femur just anterior and inferior to the origin of the lateral collateral ligament (Figure 3–6). It also receives fibers from the arcuate popliteal ligament (from the fibula head to the posterior tibia and posterior capsule) and the lateral meniscus. From its

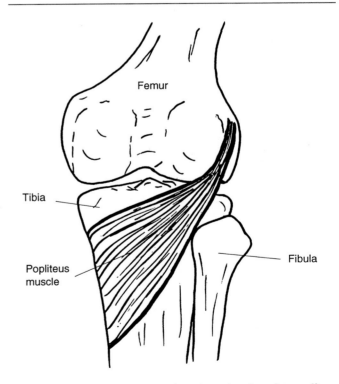

Figure 3–6 Right knee, posterior view showing the popliteus muscle.

origin, it passes under the lateral collateral ligament and forms the floor of the popliteus fossa. It inserts into the posterior surface of the tibia. The most medial portion inserts along the soleus line, where it is easily palpated.

The popliteus initiates flexion from hyperextension.[4] With a fixed origin, contraction medially rotates the tibia and flexes the tibia on the femur. With a fixed insertion, contraction of the popliteus pulls the lateral femoral condyle and lateral meniscus posteriorly and pulls the capsular ligaments out of harm's way during flexion. The popliteus by both actions is a strong medial rotator of the tibia on the femur. Normal muscle tone prevents total dependence on ligaments in hyperextension, allowing an "end feel" upon springing of the relaxed leg.

With weight bearing, the popliteus is a major stabilizer of the lateral knee. Some studies show the popliteus securing the lateral knee even with the lateral collateral ligament severed. By its posterior pull on the lateral femoral condyle, in crouching it is believed to assist the posterior cruciate ligament in preventing anterior slippage of the femur.

With a loss of normal muscle tone or strength, a patient in the erect posture will appear to have a slightly hyperextended knee. In the supine posture the affected knee will dip into greater hyperextension when relaxed than the normal knee and will have a loss of the normal "end feel."

As with the VMO, postural distortions producing an increase in the Q angle and a valgus knee place great stress on the popliteus muscle. With a loss of muscle tone and/or stretching, a persistent lateral rotation of the tibia on the femur is the usual finding.

The nerve supply is the tibial nerve (L-4, L-5, and S-1).

One of the signs of gallbladder dysfunction may be a popliteus muscle that fails to function up to its normal strength[5] (see Appendix A). The specific area to adjust if the gallbladder is involved is T4–5.

To test the popliteus, flex the knee to approximately 120°, diminishing the medial hamstring support (Figure 3–7A). Place the foot in medial rotation, and instruct the patient to hold it there. Do not have the patient medially rotate the foot (patients often will medially rotate and invert the foot, bringing into play the anterior tibialis muscle). With the patient holding, attempt lateral rotation of the foot while supporting the heel (Figure 3–7B). Do not use the toes for a contact; use a broad contact.

A common error is to test with the knee at 90°. With a popliteus weakness, the semitendinosus muscle will often be recruited for the test. Flexion beyond 90° prevents the hamstring recruitment.

Iliotibial Tract

The deep fascia begins with an attachment to the superior ramus of the pubis, inguinal ligament, iliac crest, sacrum, coccyx, sacrotuberous ligament, and ischial tuberosity. It envel-

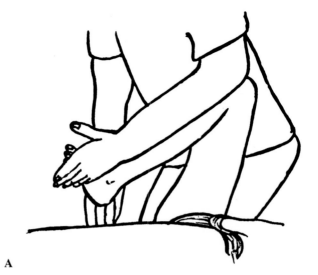

A

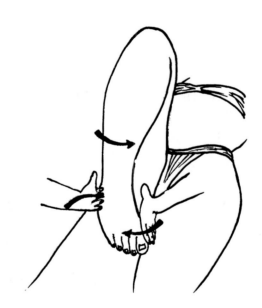

B

Figure 3–7 (A) Contacts to test the popliteus muscle. (B) Popliteus muscle test.

ops the gluteal region and the thigh with the thickest fibers along the anterior lateral thigh (fascia lata).

The fascia lata receives fibers from the tensor fascia lata muscle anteriorly and from the gluteus maximus muscle posteriorly. Passing as a broad, thick band (iliotibial tract), it has a broad insertion into all the exposed bone structures of the knee. Its insertion includes the fibula, patella, and condyle of the femur and a strong attachment to the lateral condyle of the tibia.[2]

During flexion of the knee, the fibers inserting into the tibial condyle move posteriorly on the femoral condyle, returning anteriorly with extension. The movement over the lateral condyle is sometimes the site of irritation.

Action of the iliotibial tract, influenced by the tensor fascia lata and the gluteus maximus muscles, assists in extending the knee. After flexion is initiated, it becomes a flexor of the knee and a lateral rotator of the tibia. Through the iliotibial tract, the gluteus maximus and tensor fascia lata muscles assist in stabilizing the knee.

The broad expanse of the gluteus maximus muscle and its strength prevent its testing as an indicator of its influence on the knee. Its action of stabilizing the tract is only a small part of its overall function and strength.

The tensor fascia lata muscle arises from the lateral iliac crest and the anterosuperior iliac spine. Fibers of the muscle vary in length, with some reaching the level of the lateral femoral condyle, where they join the majority of the fibers attaching to the iliotibial tract.

To test the tensor fascia lata muscle, place the patient in the supine position, elevate the extended leg to 45°, and internally rotate and abduct the leg to approximately 15° (Figure 3–8). Have the patient hold the position while applying pressure with an open hand on the ankle toward the opposite ankle. As discussed above, the gluteus maximus fixes the tract and may influence the test.

Weakness of the gluteus maximus, abdominal muscles, and quadratus lumborum allowing the ilium to move anteriorly during the test will affect the outcome. In the presence of a weak tensor fascia lata, the patient may react by posteriorly rotating the ilium to compensate; hence the importance of observation.

The nerve supply to the iliotibial tract is the superior gluteal nerve (L-4 and L-5).

Hamstrings

All three of the hamstring muscles arise from the ischial tuberosity (Figure 3–9). The long head of the biceps also has

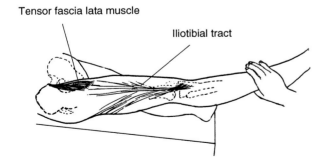

Figure 3–8 Right leg, lateral view showing the tensor fascia lata and the iliotibial tract.

Tensor fascia lata muscle

Iliotibial tract

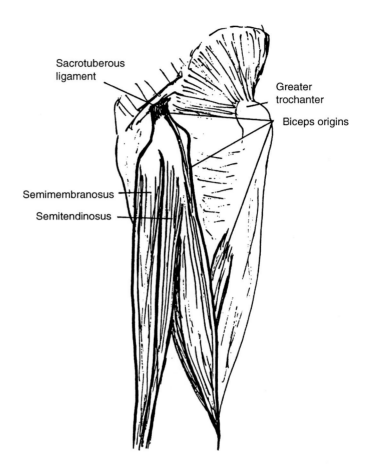

Figure 3–9 Right leg, posterior view showing the hamstring muscles.

Sacrotuberous ligament

Greater trochanter

Biceps origins

Semimembranosus

Semitendinosus

fibers to the sacrotuberous ligament. The muscle fibers blend with each other for a short distance below the origin before dividing.

The semitendinosus tendon forms the medial border of the popliteal fossa on its way to its insertion into the pes anserinus on the tibia.

The semimembranosus lies deep to the semitendinosus and inserts into a tubercle on the posterior surface of the medial tibial condyle. It also gives off some slips to the popliteal fascia and some to the oblique popliteal ligament.

The short head of the biceps femoris originates on the posterior surface of the femur as high as the lower fibers of the gluteus maximus. The long head originates on the ischial tuberosity with some fibers to the sacrotuberous ligament. The two heads blend into a common tendon that forms the lateral border of the popliteal fossa. The main part of the tendon splits and inserts on the head of the fibula on either side of the lateral collateral ligament. Some fibers of the tendon insert into the lateral collateral ligament and the lateral condyle of the tibia.

Acting together, the hamstrings flex the knee and extend the hip. The biceps with the knee flexed is a lateral rotator of the tibia. The medial hamstrings with the knee flexed are medial rotators of the tibia.

The hamstrings become posterior rotators of the pelvis only if the pelvis is flexed forward, assisting in returning to neutral. In the erect posture the hamstrings' effect on rotation of the pelvis is minimal, otherwise the large number of short hamstrings found in practice would produce a predominance of posteriorly rotated pelves, which is not the case.

The hamstrings act as stabilizers of the pelvis in the erect posture and assist in moving the pelvis from side to side.

Action of the biceps pulls the fibula proximally in the extended knee. During the first stages of flexion, its pull influences the fibula head posteriorly as well until 90° of flexion is reached, where the pull is posterior only.

The biceps' action on the fibula becomes an important factor not only in knee problems but in problems of the foot and ankle as well. The reverse is also important, with foot and ankle problems affecting biceps function.

The nerve supply for all three hamstring muscles is the sciatic nerve (L-5, S-1, and S-2).

With the patient prone, test first with the knee at 90° (Figure 3–10). With the support hand, contact the belly of the muscles while pressure is applied using the back of the wrist or an open hand.

If a muscle spasm should occur during the test, cease all pressure, and instruct the patient to relax. Straighten the leg, and apply steady pressure laterally to stretch the hamstring muscles until the spasm is over. Do not retest.

Testing may be performed at different degrees from 45° to 90° (Figure 3–11). Each places different stress on the meniscus and other structures and may help in making the diagnosis.

To emphasize the medial hamstrings, medially rotate the thigh (move the foot laterally; Figure 3–12). This brings up the medial hamstrings so that they are more prominent and may be tested with less influence from the biceps. To emphasize the lateral hamstring, move the foot medially (Figure 3–13).

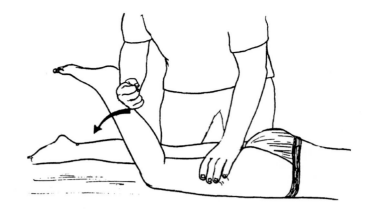

Figure 3–11 Hamstring muscle test in 80° of flexion.

Gastrocnemius and Plantaris

Both these muscles must be considered together because they have a common insertion into the calcaneus tendon. The plantaris muscle has little influence and is best considered a slip of the lateral head of the gastrocnemius origin (Figure 3–14).

The primary action of the gastrocnemius and the plantaris is plantar flexion of the ankle. The effect on the knee in the erect posture is stabilization; these muscles have little or no effect in flexion except when the ankle is dorsiflexed.

A shortened or contracted gastrocnemius may slightly flex the knee with the ankle in dorsiflexion. It would greatly restrict dorsiflexion of the ankle, however, which would be easier to recognize.

The plantaris muscle is a small muscle that may be palpated in the popliteal fossa just medial to the lateral head of the gastrocnemius. It has been the author's experience that, in some cases of hamstring weakness, deep massage of the plantaris results in a greater response by the hamstrings. The plantaris

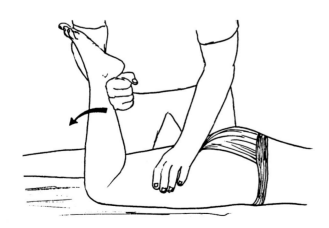

Figure 3–10 Hamstring muscle test.

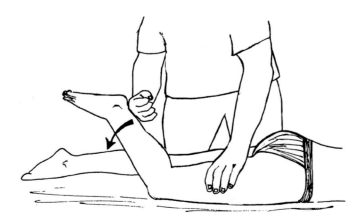

Figure 3–12 Medial hamstring muscle test with the femur rotated medially (foot moved laterally).

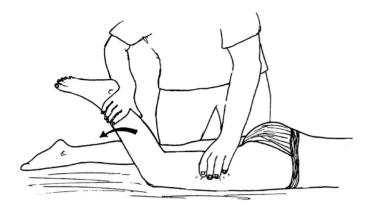

Figure 3–13 Lateral hamstring muscle test with the femur rotated laterally (foot moved medially).

may help in stabilization during flexion of the knee because some of its fibers insert into the flexor retinaculum.

The nerve supply to both muscles is the tibial nerve (S-1 and S-2).

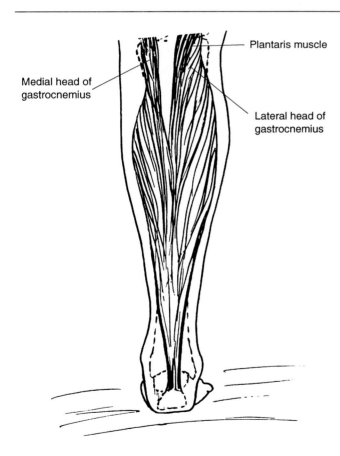

Figure 3–14 Right leg, posterior view showing plantaris and gastrocnemius muscles.

Plantaris muscle

Medial head of gastrocnemius

Lateral head of gastrocnemius

The following will test the gastrocnemius, soleus, plantaris, and, to some degree, the posterior tibialis and flexor hallucis longus. Place the patient supine, grasp the heel with the forefoot on the forearm, and attempt dorsiflexion with the patient maintaining a neutral position (Figure 3–15).

The soleus and posterior tibialis muscles may be isolated to some degree by flexing the knee, thereby removing the effect of the gastrocnemius and plantaris (Figure 3–16). The gastrocnemius and plantaris cannot be isolated. The best information to be obtained is found by testing for muscle tone and length and through palpation.

MUSCLE BALANCE

The musculoskeletal system may function within reason without great strength. The 92-lb woman who has never participated in strenuous physical activity may be completely free of pain and discomfort. She may also move through the full range of motion and be perfectly balanced even though all her muscles are weak. On the other hand, the 200-lb male bodybuilder who works out every day and whose muscles all test strong may have limited range of motion, muscle imbalance, distortion, and pain.

Imbalance is relatively easy to detect when a muscle tests weak on one side and strong on the opposite side. When both muscles test up to what is expected, the examiner must consider the possibility that, if tested to their total capacity, one may test to a greater capacity than the other. Thus an imbalance exists and must be dealt with.

If a muscle is suspected of being stretched and not functioning efficiently, it may be tested and then retested while the examiner gives manual support to the muscle (see Figure 3–3). If a positive response is found, repeat again without the support. If it is still affected, treatment with exercise and/or support may be used to restore the muscle to normal function.

A knowledge of muscle function allows the examiner to recognize imbalance by body part position, differences in the

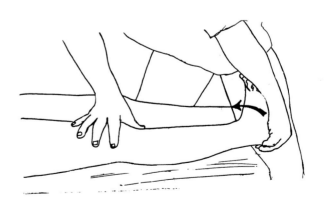

Figure 3–15 Test for gastrocnemius, plantaris, and soleus muscles.

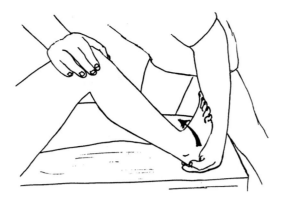

Figure 3–16 Test removing some gastrocnemius function.

range of motion, and passive stretching to test muscle tone. For example, a low shoulder with suspected weakness of the upper trapezius muscle in the sitting position may be verified with the patient supine. By pulling inferiorly on the clavicle and scapula, the true muscle length and tone may be checked

without any compensatory alterations of position due to weight bearing.

SUMMARY

Muscle testing is fraught with many variables, as indicated earlier in this chapter. When used in conjunction with observation and as a part of the overall examination, however, it is helpful in diagnosing problems. Muscles that test weak help in establishing a treatment program and in demonstrating to the patient the weaknesses. If exercises are needed, muscle testing helps persuade the patient to do them.

Fixations may produce muscle reactions, and muscle imbalance may produce fixations. When a fixation is persistent, returning repeatedly, it is necessary for the practitioner to know which muscles allow the fixation to occur as well as which muscles may produce the fixation. This information helps in initiating a program of treatment to prevent the fixation from recurring. It also improves the overall knowledge of the practitioner in how that particular articulation fits into the overall postural function.

REFERENCES

1. Kendall FP. *Muscles, Testing and Function.* New York: Churchill Livingstone; 1977.

2. Warwick R, Williams P. *Gray's Anatomy.* 35th British ed. Philadelphia: Saunders; 1973.

3. Hoppenfeld S. *Physical Examination of the Spine and Extremities.* New York: Appleton-Century-Crofts; 1976.

4. Kapandji IA. *The Physiology of the Joints.* New York: Churchill Livingstone; 1977.

5. Goodheart G. Applied Kinesiology Notes. Presented at Applied Kinesiology Seminars; 1972-1976.

Chapter 4

Imaging

Lindsay J. Rowe, MAppSc (Chiropractic),
MD, DACBR (USA), FCCR (CAN),
FACCR (AUST), FICC

This chapter reviews imaging of the most common abnormalities of the knee. Available imaging modalities are numerous, and many are utilized in the detection of specific disorders (Table 4–1).

IMAGING METHODS

Plain Film Radiography

Minimum Study

Conventional radiography remains a pivotal imaging examination in knee disorders. It is readily available, fast, and cost effective. It is standard procedure that views are obtained in both frontal and lateral planes with supplemental views as considered appropriate. The basic knee series comprises anteroposterior (AP), AP tunnel, lateral, and patellofemoral ("skyline" or tangential) views.

Technical Considerations

In general, radiographs of the knee should be obtained with a grid, although in young patients or in the case of measurements less than 10 cm this can be disregarded. An optimum exposure is in the range 55 to 60 kVp. Fine-detail or single-emulsion extremity screens and films should be utilized.

Anteroposterior View

Patient Position. This view can be obtained with the patient upright or recumbent. Upright weight-bearing views are preferable and should be obtained bilaterally with a single exposure.[1,2] Some clinicians prefer a view with the patient standing

Table 4–1 Clinical–Imaging Correlations in the Knee*

Technique	Bone Disease	Joint Disease	Soft Tissue Disease
Plain film radiography	+++	+++	+
Computed tomography	++++	+++	+++
Magnetic resonance imaging	+++	++++	+++++
Bone scan	+++++	++	+++
Arthrography	+	++	+
Ultrasound	–	+	+++

* This rating scale is based on the approximate clinical usefulness of a given imaging method in a particular clinical circumstance. For example, note that in bone disease nuclear scans are particularly sensitive, as is computed tomography. Conversely, observe that ultrasound offers little value in bone disorders. All modalities are assessed on a scale of 0 (–) to 5 (+++++).

on one leg to prevent support from the uninvolved leg (stork view).[3] With recumbent films the limb is internally rotated approximately 5° with the ankle stabilized by a suitably placed sandbag across the lower leg.

Tube Position. Cephalad tube angulation of 5° with the central ray centered 1 cm below the patellar inferior pole is optimum. This facilitates the beam passing parallel to the articular surface of the tibial plateau.

Application. The osseous components of the distal femur, proximal tibia, and fibula along with the patella can all be identified (Figure 4–1). This view is especially valuable in the assessment of the femorotibial joint compartment, which should be no smaller than 5 mm. This is further enhanced

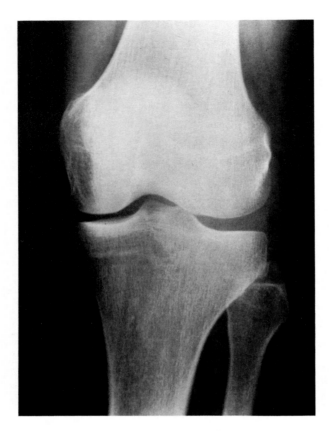

Figure 4-1 AP view. In this standard projection the bony structures of the femur, tibia, and fibula are well demonstrated. Note also that the femorotibial joint space is clearly seen. The patella, however, is obscured. *Comment*: This view should be obtained in weight bearing to show loss of joint space and the presence of lateral tibial shift, changes in a degenerative knee joint that are not adequately demonstrated on recumbent views.

when the projection is obtained in the upright position. Although the patella is obscured by the femur, it is in this view that any fracture lines or bipartite anomalies can often be identified.

Anteroposterior Intercondylar (Tunnel) View

Patient Position. The patient can be prone with the knee flexed to 45°. Alternatively, an easier position is with the patient kneeling and leaning forward to position the joint at 45°.[4]

Tube Position. The central ray is directed to the popliteal fossa through the joint. When the patient is prone, the tube is angled caudad 45°. In the kneeling position no tube angulation is required. The milliampere-seconds should be increased to at least 50% greater than that of the AP projection.

Applications. As the name implies, this is a specific view that provides additional detail on contents of the intercondylar

notch, especially loose bodies and tibial eminences, and exposes more of the femoral condylar surfaces[5] (Figure 4-2).

Lateral View

Patient Position. The patient lies with the study side down and the knee flexed to 45°. The upper leg is carried forward and placed on the table to assist stability. The central ray is 2 cm distal to the medial epicondyle with the long axis of the femur coincident with the vertical component of the beam.

Tube Position. Some clinicians advocate the use of 5° of cephalad tube tilt to assist in superimposing both femoral condyles.

Applications. The patella and patellofemoral joint space are well demonstrated in this view. Additionally, the femoral and

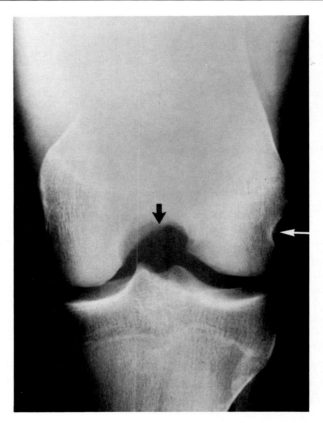

Figure 4-2 AP intercondylar (tunnel) view. With the knee flexed, the intercondylar notch comes into profile (black arrow). In addition, the tibial eminences are clearly displayed, and another tangential view of the femoral condyles is obtained. Note that the groove for the popliteus tendon (normal variant) is prominent (white arrow); it should not be mistaken for an erosive process. *Comment*: This projection may show loose bodies and other abnormalities in the notch that are not visible on the standard AP view. Osteochondritis dissecans and Spontaneous Osteonecrosis of the Knee (SONK) also may be seen only on this view.

tibial components, tibial tuberosity, and posterior joint compartment are depicted (Figure 4–3). To demonstrate better the tibial tuberosity and adjacent soft tissues, such as in the assessment of Osgood-Schlatter disease, the tibia should be rotated internally by 5° and the exposure reduced by at least 50%.[6] A cross-table lateral view with the patient supine is especially useful in demonstrating fat–fluid levels as a sign of an intraarticular fracture where there has been release of medullary bone fat into the joint cavity.

Patellofemoral (Sunrise, Skyline, or Tangential) View

Patient Position. The patient is prone with the knee flexed to more than 90°. A strap may be employed to assist in stabilizing the limb during the exposure.

Tube Position. The central ray is directed beneath the patella through the patellofemoral joint with tight collimation.

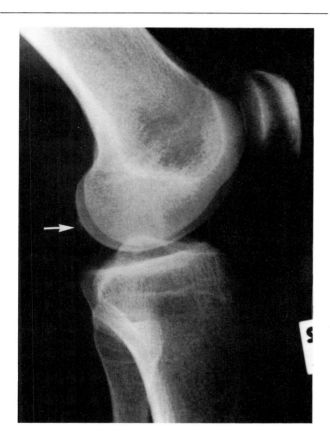

Figure 4–3 Lateral view. All bones are seen in a different profile. Note the clear presentation of the patella and the patellofemoral joint. The fibula head normally overlaps the proximal tibia. *Comment:* The fabella (normal variant) lies above the joint line just behind the femoral condyles (arrow). Observe the clearly defined loss of bone density in the distal femur, which is due to the intercondylar notch (Ludloff's fleck).

Applications. This is the optimum view to depict the patella surfaces, patella alignment, and patellofemoral joint[7] (Figure 4–4).

Alternative Patellofemoral Joint Views

Various techniques have been described in the adequate assessment of the patellofemoral joint because the traditional projection described above with the knee so flexed does not accurately assess patella subluxation, which characteristically occurs in lesser degrees of flexion. Because the tube position in all views can potentially expose the pelvic area, a lead apron suitably positioned should be employed. At least four other variations have been advocated:

1. Hughston view: The patient is prone, the leg is flexed 50° to 60°, and the tube is angled toward the head parallel to the plane of the patellofemoral joint.[8]
2. Knutsson view: The patient is supine with the knee flexed and the tube horizontal. This requires a special film holder.[9]
3. Merchant view: The patient is supine with the knee flexed 45° over the table edge and the tube angled toward the feet. A special film holder is required.[10]
4. Inferosuperior view (reversed Merchant view): The patient is supine with the knee flexed over the table edge. The beam is angled up toward the head, and the patient holds the film perpendicular to the central ray.[11]

Stress View

Patient Position. The patient is supine with the leg extended. This view is best performed under general anesthesia to fully evaluate ligamentous integrity. Valgus stress is applied across the joint.

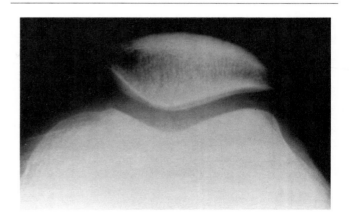

Figure 4–4 Normal patellofemoral (skyline) projection. Observe the congruence of the joint surface and how the patella apex lies within the intercondylar groove. *Comment:* This view is especially useful in the depiction of the patellofemoral joint, patella, and femoral condyles.

Tube Position. The tube is angled perpendicular to the knee.

Applications. This view is an attempt to assess the degree of disruption of the collateral ligaments. The key sign is joint space widening.

Arthrography

Technique

The joint is aspirated, and 2 to 5 mL of water-soluble contrast medium and 30 mL of air are injected. The knee is then flexed and extended a number of times. Under fluoroscopy, 6 to 12 exposures of each meniscus are made with increasing rotation. Traction and varus or valgus stress are also applied. At the end of the procedure, AP and lateral films are taken for cruciate ligament analysis and to search for evidence of Baker's cyst.

Applications

Arthrography has been the traditional diagnostic method for the evaluation of intraarticular pathology. The accuracy for the diagnosis of meniscal tears approaches 99% for medial tears and 93% for lateral tears.[12] Cruciate ligament tears are less reliably diagnosed. Accurate assessment depends on the use of proper technique, with accuracy ranging from 50% to 90%.[12] Other conditions for which arthrography may be of use are chondromalacia patellae, osteochondritis dissecans, loose bodies, and pigmented villonodular synovitis. Abnormal extension of contrast material into a bone–prosthesis interface can be used to detect loosening.

Computed Tomography

Technique

With computed tomography (CT), images must be obtained sequentially with a 10-mm slice thickness or less. Soft tissue windows are used to display muscle and periarticular detail. Bone windows are used to demonstrate skeletal abnormalities.

Applications

CT of the knee as a diagnostic tool has not found wide acceptance for diagnosing intraarticular or periarticular abnormalities. This is due to the lack of tissue differentiation and resolution in structures such as menisci and ligaments. Three-dimensional reconstruction may have some application in cruciate ligament abnormalities.[13] The major application of knee CT has been in the assessment of tumors, infections, and fractures.[14]

Magnetic Resonance Imaging

Technique

The standard magnetic resonance (MR) examination of the knee is performed with the patient supine and the affected knee in 10° to 20° of external rotation and full extension, a position that optimizes visualization of the anterior cruciate ligament. It is essential that both coronal and sagittal sequences be performed on all patients. Both T1- and T2-weighted images are obtained. Ligaments and menisci show as black structures (low signal intensity). For meniscal assessment, a narrow window (meniscal window) is used to demonstrate more fully intrameniscal detail. Intraarticular effusions are best depicted on T2-weighted images, where fluid becomes white (high signal intensity).

Applications

In many centers MR imaging has replaced knee arthrography. This depends largely on availability.

The advantages of MR imaging include its noninvasive nature, lack of known side effects, lack of ionizing radiation, ability to image in any plane, and lack of operator dependence. MR imaging is capable of diagnosing and evaluating intraarticular (menisci and cruciate ligaments), periarticular (neoplasms and collateral ligaments), and subchondral abnormalities (stress fractures and osteonecrosis) as well as lesions that are not accessible to the arthroscopist.[15]

Isotopic Bone Scan

Technique

The two most common agents employed are ^{99m}Tc and ^{67}Ga. Essentially, the radionuclide is injected intravenously and becomes protein bound, whereupon it perfuses into skeletal sites and binds to the bone crystal surface. Radionuclide that is not incorporated into bone is renally excreted; excretion may be as high as 50% 1 hour after injection.[16] As the isotope undergoes degeneration, γ rays are emitted, which are detected by a scintillation camera. The greater the bone turnover, the higher the concentration of isotope and the greater the scintillation count, which produces the hot spot on the resultant image.

Three studies are usually obtained after injection (three-phase study). One obtained immediately depicts the vascular tree distally and is called a flow study. Within 5 minutes, images depict the capillary and venous phases of perfusion; these are called a blood pool study. At around 2 to 3 hours, there is significant bone uptake for the bone image study.

Applications

Nuclear imaging is an extremely sensitive marker of bone and joint disease. It has high sensitivity but relatively low specificity. Any disease process that disturbs the normal balance of bone production and resorption can be depicted on bone scan, usually as an area of increased uptake (hot spot) or occasionally decreased uptake (cold spot). Increased bone uptake can be demonstrated with only a 3% to 5% change in bone activity; therefore, this type of study is especially useful in the early depiction of infections, tumors, stress fractures, avascular necrosis, articular disorders, and bone pain of undetermined etiology. It should be noted, however, that there will be an increased uptake in normal structures, such as developing growth plates and adult metaphyses.

MEASUREMENTS OF THE KNEE

Patella Position

Vertical Alignment

On a lateral view the length of the patella is compared with the length of the patella ligament (Figure 4–5). These measurements are generally equal; normal variation does not exceed 20%.[17] If the patella is excessively high, this is called patella alta and may predispose to patella subluxation, patella dislocation, or chondromalacia patellae. A low-riding patella (patella baja) may be seen in polio, achondroplasia, juvenile rheumatoid arthritis, and tibial tubercle transposition.

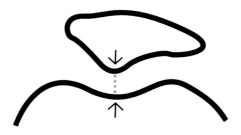

Figure 4–6 Patella apex sign. The patella is in correct alignment when its apex lies directly above the deepest section of the intercondylar sulcus. *Comment*: This is a useful visual clue in the detection of subtle subluxations of the patellofemoral joint.

Patella Apex

The patella is centered when its apex is directly above the deepest section of the intercondylar sulcus[3](Figure 4–6).

Sulcus Angle

Lines drawn from the highest points on the medial and lateral condyles to the lowest point of the intercondylar sulcus form an angle (Figure 4–7). Normally this angle should be 138° (range 132° to 144°).[3,10] Greater measurements (shallow intercondylar groove) predispose to subluxation and dislocation.

Lateral Patellofemoral Angle

A line tangential to the femoral condyles is intersected by a line joining the limits of the lateral facet[11] (Figure 4–8). The angle is normally open. In patellar subluxation, these lines are parallel or open medially.

Lateral Patellofemoral Joint Index

The narrowest medial joint space measurement is divided by the narrowest lateral joint space measurement (Figure 4–9).

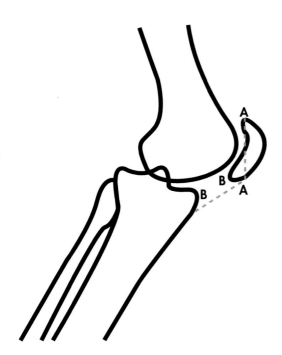

Figure 4–5 Vertical patella alignment. The length of the patella is measured from pole to pole (A–A). The patellar tendon is measured on its deep surface from the lower pole to its attachment on the tibial tubercle (B–B). *Comment*: Normally these measurements are equal, although the range of normal is 20% variation. A high-riding patella (patella alta) or a low-riding patella (patella baja) can be determined from this measurement.

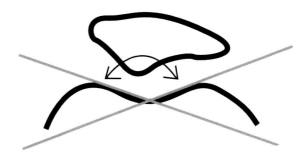

Figure 4–7 Sulcus angle. Two lines are drawn tangential to the medial and lateral condylar surfaces to the lowest point of the intercondylar sulcus. *Comment*: Normally this measurement is 138° (range 132° to 144°). A shallow groove (>144°) may predispose to subluxation and dislocation.

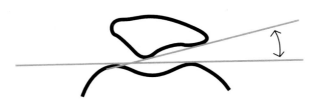

Figure 4–8 Lateral patellofemoral angle. Tangential lines are drawn through the femoral condyles and the lateral patella. Normally these form an open angle on the lateral side. *Comment*: In patellar subluxation these lines are parallel, or the angle is open medially.

This index is normally less than or equal to 1.0. A value greater than 1.0 is noted in patients with chondromalacia patellae.[11]

Lateral Patellar Displacement

A line is drawn tangential to the medial and lateral condylar surfaces (Figure 4–10). A perpendicular line at the medial edge of the femoral condyle normally lies 1 mm medial to the patella or closer.[11]

Varus–Valgus Angulation

On the AP standing film, lines are drawn along the femoral and tibial shafts and normally intersect to form an angle of 5° to 7°.[3] This angle is greater than 7° in genu valgus and less than 5° in genu varus (Figure 4–11).

Lateral Tibial Subluxation

Normally the femoral and tibial shaft lines intersect at the knee joint. If the lines intersect above the joint line, lateral tibial subluxation is present.[3] This displacement can be quantified by measuring the distance between parallel lines drawn on the most lateral surfaces of the femur and tibia[18] (Figure 4–12).

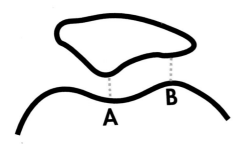

Figure 4–9 Lateral patellofemoral joint index. This index is the ratio between the narrowest medial joint space (A) and the narrowest lateral joint space (B). *Comment*: The index is normally 1.0 or less. An index greater than 1.0 may denote chondromalacia patellae or degenerative joint disease.

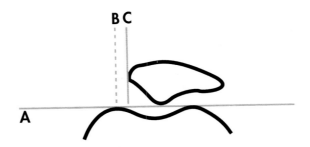

Figure 4–10 Lateral patellar displacement. A line is drawn tangentially through the femoral condyles (A–A). A line perpendicular to A–A is drawn at the medial edge of the medial condyle (B–A). Another perpendicular line is drawn at the medial edge of the patella (C–A). Measurement is made between lines B–A and C–A. *Comment*: Normally the B–C interval is less than 1 mm. Measurements greater than 1 mm indicate patellar subluxation or dislocation.

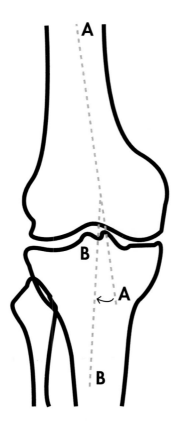

Figure 4–11 Varus–valgus angulation. On an upright AP view, lines are drawn through the femoral and tibial shafts (A–A and B–B, respectively). These intersect at or below the joint to form an angle inferiorly. *Comment*: The normal value is between 5° and 7°; measurements greater than 7° indicate genu valgus, and measurements less then 5° indicate genu varus. Furthermore, if these lines intersect above the joint, lateral displacement of the tibia is usually present.

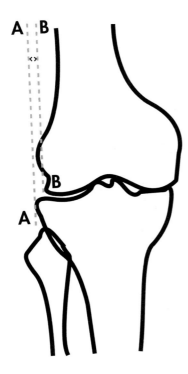

Figure 4–12 Lateral tibial subluxation. The distance between the lateral margins of the femur and tibia is determined by drawing vertical lines tangential to their lateral margins (A–A and B–B, respectively). *Comment*: The amount of lateral tibial displacement can be quantified and indicates degenerative joint disease causing ligamentous laxity. This measurement is best applied in weight-bearing studies.

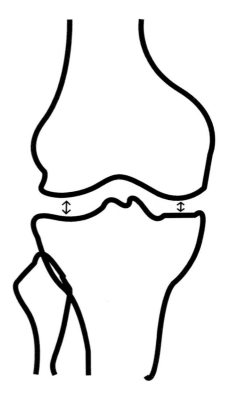

Figure 4–13 Femorotibial joint space. On weight-bearing studies, the medial and lateral femorotibial joint spaces are measured at their narrowest dimensions. *Comment*: The normal range is between 5 and 11 mm. Narrowed joint spaces are indicative of joint disease, and widening may indicate acromegaly.

Femorotibial Joint Space

On standing views the cartilage space is 5 to 11 mm in thickness[1] (Figure 4–13).

Axial Relations

Femoral Angle

Lines are drawn through the axis of the femoral shaft and tangential to the femoral condyles (Figure 4–14). The angle on the lateral side is measured; it ranges from 75° to 85°. This measurement is useful is assessing postfracture deformities and overgrowth or hypoplasia of the femoral condyles.[19]

Tibial Angle

Lines are drawn through the axis of the tibial shaft and tangential to the tibial condyles (Figure 4–14). The angle on the lateral side is measured; it ranges from 85° to 100°. This measurement is useful in assessing postfracture deformities and overgrowth or hypoplasia of the tibial plateau.[19]

Tibial Plateau Angle

The angle of the tibial plateau is defined on the lateral view by three lines: a line tangential to the anterior tibial cortex, a line tangential to the plateau, and a line perpendicular to the cortex line. The angle between the latter of these two lines is measured; it varies between 5° and 20° with an average of 15° (Figure 4–15). This measurement is useful in determining the degree of depression in tibial plateau fractures.[19]

Femoral Condyle Position

On a lateral view, one line is drawn along the anterior femoral cortex and another through the intercondylar cortex (Blumensaat's line). The angle between these lines averages 34° and helps quantify the deformity from supracondylar fracture[20] (Figure 4–16).

Sagittal Instability

A preliminary lateral non–weight-bearing film with at least 15° of flexion is obtained. A second upright weight-bearing film in at least 15° of flexion is required. A line is drawn tangential to the tibial articular surface, and a second perpendicular line is drawn upward with the distance to the posterior femoral condylar surface measured. This is done on both lateral views, and the measurements are compared. Comparison bilaterally with the normal knee is desirable. In general, the

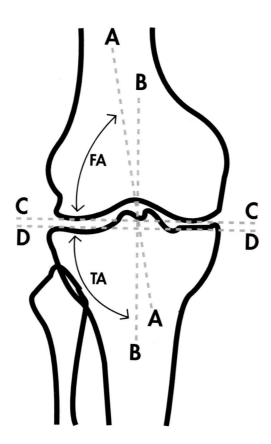

Figure 4–14 Axial relations. Lines are drawn through the femoral and tibial shafts (A–A and B–B, respectively) and tangential to the femoral and tibial condyles (C–C and D–D, respectively). The femoral angle (FA) ranges from 75° to 85°. The tibial angle (TA) ranges from 85° to 100°. *Comment*: These lines and angles are useful in the quantification of condylar or shaft deformities.

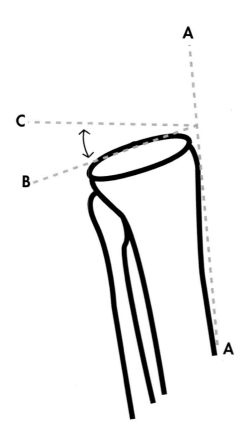

Figure 4–15 Tibial plateau angle. On the lateral film three lines are drawn: tangential to the tibial anterior cortex (A–A), tangential to the tibial plateau (A–B), and perpendicular to A–A (A–C). The angle between A–B and A–C is the tibial plateau angle. *Comment*: This angle usually ranges between 5° and 20° (average, 15°). In plateau fractures the amount of depression can be quantified.

difference between erect and recumbent films is less than 3 mm, with larger measurements indicating increasing cruciate insufficiency[21] (Figure 4–17).

CONGENITAL ANOMALIES AND VARIANTS

Bone Islands (Enostoma)

Clinical Features

Bone islands are histologically normal compact bone lying within the medullary cavity. They are clinically insignificant skeletal variants that require differentiation from osteoid osteoma, Brodie's abscess, and osteoblastic metastasis. Serum alkaline phosphatase is normal with bone islands. Change in size with time is common in up to one third of bone islands.[22,23]

Imaging Features

On conventional radiographs a bone island is recognizable as a round to oval, homogeneously sclerotic focus lying within the epiphysis or metaphysis (Figure 4–18). Occasionally

they may exist as more elongated forms, usually with their long axis oriented along trabecular lines. They are never diaphyseal, nor is any periosteal reaction evident. Intermittently some cases will demonstrate a spiculated brush border due to thickened trabeculae that abut the lesion. A few may coexist simultaneously, but if they are numerous, symmetric, and found at other long bone metaphyses, then this is most likely due to osteopoikilosis.

Bone islands on bone scan may demonstrate isotope uptake.[24] CT scan is useful to determine whether there is a contained radiolucent area, which would be consistent with osteoid osteoma or Brodie's abscess.

Fabella (Sesamoid Bone of the Gastrocnemius)

Clinical Features

The fabella is a sesamoid bone that lies within the tendon of the lateral head of the gastrocnemius muscle. It is a normal skeletal variant of no clinical significance, but it must not be

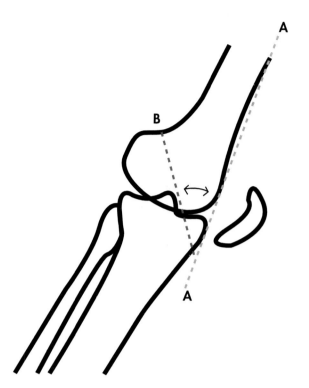

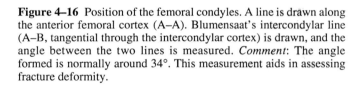

Figure 4–16 Position of the femoral condyles. A line is drawn along the anterior femoral cortex (A–A). Blumensaat's intercondylar line (A–B, tangential through the intercondylar cortex) is drawn, and the angle between the two lines is measured. *Comment*: The angle formed is normally around 34°. This measurement aids in assessing fracture deformity.

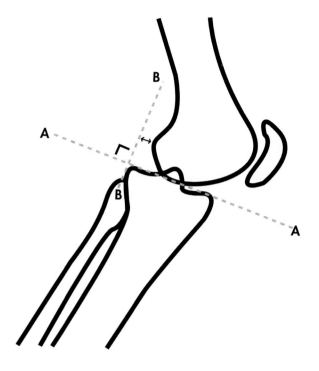

Figure 4–17 Sagittal instability. A line is drawn tangential to the tibial plateau (A–A). A line perpendicular to A–A is drawn through the posterior tibial articular surface (B–B). The distance from line B–B to the posterior surface of the femoral condyle is measured. *Comment*: These measurements must be compared with those on a weight-bearing film. A difference of more than 3 mm may be indicative of instability, although comparisons with the other (unaffected) knee are more meaningful.

confused with a bone fragment from fracture, osteochondritis dissecans, or synoviochondrometaplasia. It occurs in up to 20% of the population.[25]

Imaging Features

On conventional radiographs the fabella lies in the posterior and lateral aspects of the knee (see Figure 4–3). On the frontal view it characteristically lies above the joint cavity and can be seen superimposed on the lateral condyle. It can be of variable shape, from round and smooth to triangular. It is bilateral in more than 85% of cases.[25] In advanced osteoarthritis of the knee, osteophytes and cystic changes can be seen. Avulsion of the medial head of the gastrocnemius tendon can be identified when the fabella is displaced medially and inferiorly.

Growth Arrest Lines (Harris' Lines, Park's Lines)

Clinical Features

Transverse, linear, opaque metaphyseal bands are a common radiographic variant of no clinical relevance.[25] They usually are found in the metaphyses of the distal femur and proximal and distal tibia. Less obvious expressions do occur in other bones, including the pelvis and subendplate zones of the vertebral bodies. They are thought to result from temporary cessation of skeletal growth, which may be related to severe illness. Such lines have been observed in chemotherapy for childhood diseases such as leukemia as well as in lead poisoning (lead lines). The main clinical implication is the need to identify the lines correctly and not to confuse them with stress fractures.

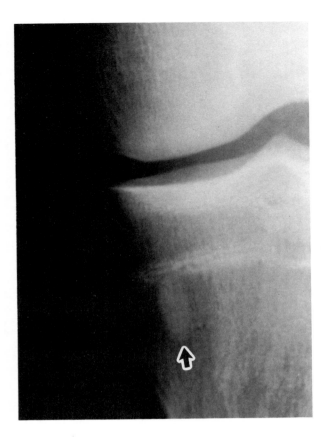

Figure 4–18 Bone island. An oval opacity is present within the tibial metaphysis (arrow). *Comment*: Bone islands around the knee are an extremely common radiographic finding of no clinical significance. They are often elongated along the orientation of trabecular lines and lack any internal lucency or periosteal response, which are useful differentiating features from osteoid osteoma or Brodie's abscess.

Imaging Features

The lines are recognizable on conventional radiographs as transverse, thin, opaque bands, typically within the metaphysis and occasionally the epiphysis. Solitary or multiple forms occur. They are bilateral and symmetric.

Segmented Patella (Bipartite/Tripartite/Multipartite/ Accessory Patella)

Clinical Features

The patella is a sesamoid bone that becomes radiographically visible at about 6 years of age. It arises from a single ossification center, but in approximately 2% to 3% of individuals this center may fragment and result in a variable number of patella segments.[26] The most common form is a small separated fragment at the superolateral pole, which is designated as a bipartite patella. These occur bilaterally in up to 40% of patients and are up to nine times more common in boys.[26–28] The majority are clinically insignificant radio-

graphic findings. There has been some suggestion that traumatic loosening of the fibrous bridge between the fragments may become a focus of pain that is unresponsive to conservative measures and is aggravated by activity.[26,29] In these unusual cases, surgical excision of the isolated fragment may be curative.

Imaging Features

The anomaly is adequately visualized on conventional radiographs. On frontal views the separated fragment is most common at the superolateral pole (Figure 4–19). The margins of the opposing segments are typically sclerotic and smooth, which readily allow exclusion of acute fracture, although in the presence of trauma this may be difficult.[30] Isotopic bone scan of a bipartite patella in symptomatic patients showing increased uptake at the separation site indicates bone activity and probably inflammation.[29]

Dorsal Defect of the Patella

Clinical Features

Virtually all cases are discovered as an incidental radiographic variant, although a causal association has been made with patella subluxation as a stress-induced anomaly at the insertion of the vastus lateralis.[31] The incidence is less than 1%, and there is no clear gender predilection.[27,32] Less than 50% occur bilaterally.[32] Histopathology of the defect has revealed necrotic bone or repair without inflammation.[32–35]

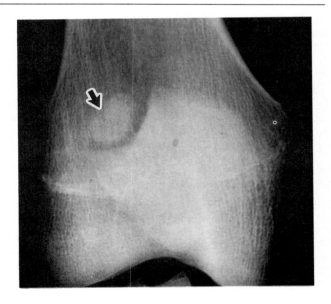

Figure 4–19 Segmented (bipartite) patella. A clearly separated segment is evident at the characteristic location of the outer upper pole of the patella (arrow). Note the smooth margins of the cleft. *Comment*: Such patellar defects can be present bilaterally in up to 40% of individuals, the majority being clinically insignificant.

Imaging Features

The defect exists as a well-defined, round lytic lesion with a sclerotic margin in the superolateral pole of the patella (Figure 4–20). The average size is 9 mm; the size ranges from 4 to 26 mm.[27,35] Bone scans may demonstrate increased uptake, and arthrography reveals intact overlying cartilage.[33] MR imaging clearly identifies the defect.[36] The major differential diagnostic considerations include osteochondritis dissecans, osteoid osteoma, and Brodie's abscess.

Tibial Tuberosity

During the adolescent phase the tibial epiphysis undergoes gradual union to the adjacent metaphysis. One or more osseous centers develop in the tibial tuberosity between 8 and 14 years which coalesce with the epiphysis and should not be confused as evidence of pathologic fragmentation such as Osgood-Schlatter disease. The cartilaginous physis can simulate a fracture.

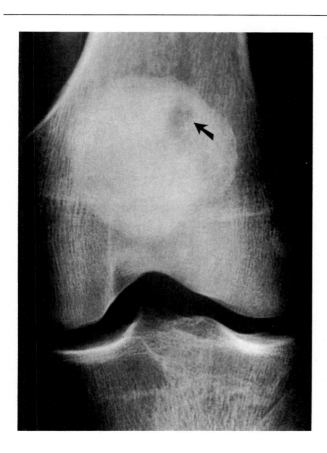

Figure 4–20 Dorsal defect of the patella. A well-defined, round, lucent defect is apparent at the outer upper pole of the patella (arrow). *Comment*: Such lesions are uncommon and of no clinical significance. Courtesy of Neil Manson, DC, Newcastle, Australia.

Vacuum Phenomenon

Occasionally a thin, waferlike radiolucency may be seen in the joint space, especially on tunnel and stress views. It is more common in the medial joint space and cannot be construed as evidence of degenerative joint disease. A vacuum within the subchondral bone of a femoral condyle is abnormal and is a sign of spontaneous osteonecrosis (SONK).

Femoral Triangle (Ludloff's Fleck)

On the lateral view a distinct lucent zone is often seen overlying the femoral epiphysis (see Figure 4–3). This is due to thin cortices of the femoral condyles.[25]

Popliteus Groove

A few millimeters above the joint line along the lateral femoral condyle, a distinct, pitlike defect is usually visible; this is the groove for the tendon of the popliteus muscle. This is often accentuated on the tunnel projection and should not be mistaken as evidence of a bony erosion[25] (see Figure 4–2).

Pseudo–Osteochondritis Dissecans

In the young individual, developmental variation in ossification of both femoral condylar articular surfaces may mimic osteochondritis dissecans. This can be seen on frontal and lateral views[37,38] (Figure 4–21).

Distal Femur Irregularity

Areas of cortical irregularity are common within the femoral metaphysis, usually at the posterior, anterior, and medial surfaces.

Posterior Surface

On lateral and oblique views, the posterior surface of the femoral metaphysis is often irregular and gives the impression of periosteal new bone (Figure 4–22). This is more common in patients younger than 20 years and is not a manifestation of an avulsive cortical lesion. It is cold on nuclear imaging.[39]

Anterior Surface

Adjacent to the anterior junction of the growth plate, localized metaphyseal cortical irregularity may be seen.[40]

Medial Surface

On frontal and oblique views, a similar irregularity may be seen at the medial metaphysis.

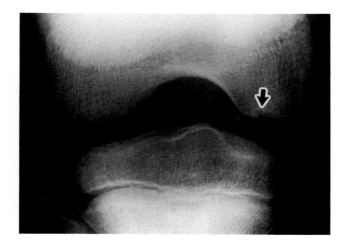

Figure 4–21 Pseudo-osteochondritis dissecans in an 8-year-old patient. Observe the apparent defect at the weight-bearing surface of the medial condyle (arrow). *Comment*: This is a common variant in ossification in patients younger than 12 years and should not be confused with osteochondritis dissecans, which in adolescents usually involves more of the intercondylar surface of the medial condyle. Courtesy of Inger F. Villadsen, DC, Newcastle, Australia.

Pseudoperiostitis

Localized areas of pseudoperiostitis are commonly seen along the fibula, tibia, and distal femur. At the tibia and fibula these are often expressions of the attachment of the interosseous membrane (Figure 4–23). Further down into the proximal diaphysis of the tibia, the soleal line may be prominent.[41]

In the mid-diaphysis of the femur, especially on its posterior surface, the linea aspera may simulate periosteal new bone. On the frontal view the linea aspera is seen as two parallel linear opacities (track sign).[42]

Fong's Syndrome

An association has been recorded between iliac horns, nail defects, and hypoplastic patellae. Synonyms include nail-patella syndrome and Hereditary Osteo-Onycho-Dysplasia (HOOD) syndrome. Other recorded findings have included clinodactyly, joint contractures, muscle hypoplasia, and renal dysplasia. At the knee, overgrowth of the medial condyle can precipitate genu valgus; the patella is prone to lateral subluxation and dislocation. Elbow anomalies involving dysplasia of the radial head are also common.

TRAUMATIC INJURIES

The knee is especially vulnerable to traumatic injuries, which can affect the osseous and soft tissue components. Soft tissue injuries are far more common than bony lesions and as

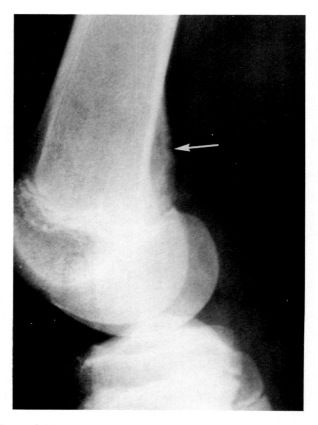

Figure 4–22 Distal femur irregularity, posterior surface (arrow). *Comment*: This is a common normal variant, especially in skeletally immature patients. This cortical irregularity simulates a destructive bone lesion.

such may require more than plain radiographs for detection. The most common defects are meniscal and ligament injuries. The most common bone to fracture at the knee is the tibial plateau.

Imaging Signs of Knee Trauma

Fracture Line

A linear radiolucency in any direction may be seen. It is often best observed at the cortical margins, where the bone is most dense. Transverse fractures are often associated with bone pathology, such as tumors. If a sclerotic, smooth margin is evident at the fracture line, nonunion and pseudoarthrosis should be suspected.

Zone of Impaction

Impaction or compressive type forces may telescope the trabeculae in the localized site, creating an area of linear opacity. In the early stages of healing, this can be further accentuated by callus and may be the only sign of an otherwise occult or stress fracture.

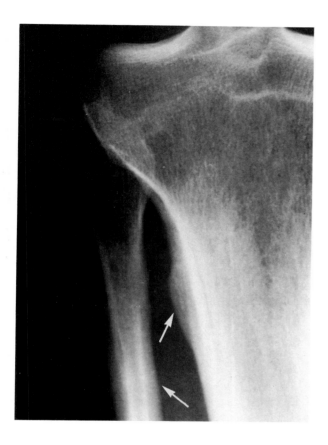

Figure 4–23 Pseudoperiostitis, tibia and fibula. Observe the localized bony density beyond the confines of the normal cortex (arrows). *Comment*: Such a finding is common at the tibia and fibula, especially at the surface, where the interosseous membrane attaches. Similarity to hypertrophic osteoarthropathy and periosteal-inducing conditions such as tumors, infections, and stress fractures can make this a confusing variant.

Fragments

Separated fragments at the fracture site are classified as comminuted fractures. An exception is where a piece of articular bone is disrupted; this is called an osteochondral fracture, of which osteochondritis dissecans constitutes an example.

Callus

At the fracture site, organization of the contained hematoma and mechanical elevation of the adjacent periosteum provoke new bone formation. This can be seen as early as 5 to 7 days after injury and persists for many weeks. It is often the only sign of an unrecognized stress fracture and, because of its proliferative appearance, can be confused with an active neoplasm, especially osteosarcoma. The callus varies in appearance from an initial veil-like pattern which progressively consolidates into a homogenous bony bridge. Any periosteal

new bone tends to be of a solid or laminated form. With remodeling, the initial fracture site may not be identifiable.

Malalignment

This can be in a transverse, longitudinal, or rotational direction. The degree of apposition should also be assessed.

Effusion

Above the patella the suprapatellar pouch can be distended on lateral views, especially when the suprapatellar fat is seen to be displaced anteriorly. A cross-table lateral view can visualize a distinct linear fluid level from released intramedullary fat secondary to an intraarticular fracture floating on a hemarthrosis (lipohemarthrosis; Figure 4–24). This is called the FBI sign (**F**at-**B**lood-**I**nterface). Gas in the soft tissues or joint may indicate a compound injury or complicating gangrene.

Osteoporosis

Marked deossification of the epiphyses and metaphyses at the joint can follow acute immobilization. Early there is distinct linear deossification in the subchondral bone. With mobilization after healing, there is rapid restitution to normal density. Care must be taken to exclude septic arthritis as a cause for such regional osteoporosis; the two can be radiographically indistinguishable.

Myositis Ossificans

Significant posttraumatic intramuscular or ligamentous hematoma may undergo organization and subsequent ossifica-

---

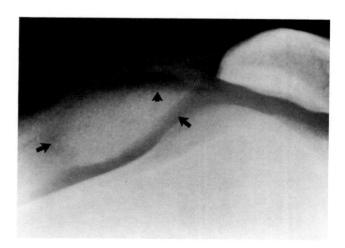

Figure 4–24 Lipohemarthrosis (FBI sign). On this cross-table lateral view, note the soft tissue density of the effusion within the suprapatellar bursa (arrows) and the discrete linear interface between blood and fat (arrowhead). *Comment*: This finding is due to an intraarticular fracture releasing fatty bone marrow into the joint cavity. Even if a fracture cannot be located, its presence is assured when this sign is seen.

tion. The earliest plain film findings can ensue within 3 to 4 weeks after the injury and may progress over the next 10 to 12 weeks. The earliest sign is a thin, wavy, calcific density separated from the adjacent bone cortex.

Fixation Artifacts

After the removal of surgical hardware used in repair of the fracture remnant, bone artifacts remain often indefinitely. These represent an electroplating-like reaction at the bone–metal interface, resulting in compact bone being deposited. This reaction is seen at the site of screws, intramedullary rods, and support stems of joint prostheses. If a gap of greater than 1 mm is present at the bone–metal interface, this can be a sign of loosening of the implant.

Degenerative Joint Disease

Posttraumatic joint deterioration can be seen radiographically, especially when complicated by malalignment, intraarticular extension, meniscal damage, significant hemarthrosis, or infection. The earliest changes are rarely seen before one year.

Fractures of the Femur

These occur above the condyles (supracondylar) or through them (condylar).

Supracondylar Fracture

The fracture line may be oblique, spiral, or transverse. Transverse fractures should raise the suspicion of underlying bone pathology. Supracondylar fractures have a strong tendency to rotate posteriorly because of the pull of the gastrocnemius.

Condylar Fracture

A Y or T configuration is commonly seen. The key feature is that these fractures are intraarticular and can be complicated by severe joint dysfunction. Occasionally a small osteochondral fragment may be displaced from the articular surface.

Fractures of the Tibia

Tibial Plateau Fracture (Bumper or Fender Fracture)

Valgus or varus forces thrust the contralateral femoral condyle into the reciprocating tibial surface, which either depresses its surface or shears the condyle away. The lateral plateau is involved in 80% of cases (Figure 4–25). There is often associated collateral ligament damage and complicating osteoarthritis.

Tibial Eminence (Spine) Fracture

These are readily overlooked because they may have minimal displacement. They are more frequent in young patients

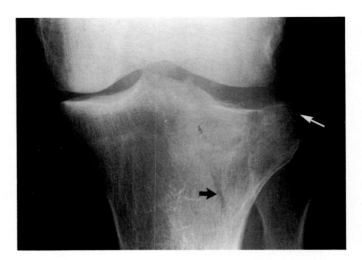

Figure 4–25 Tibial plateau (bumper) fracture. There is a subtle fracture through the lateral tibial plateau (arrows). *Comment:* The lateral plateau is involved in 80% of cases as a result of impaction of the adjacent femoral condyle, usually from a valgus-type force.

with hyperextension injuries and are associated with cruciate ligament disruption.

Avulsion of the Tibial Tuberosity

As an isolated injury, this is unusual. It should not be confused with the normal growth plate beneath the tuberosity in the young; bilateral comparison views will be helpful in these cases.

Segond's Fracture

Avulsion fracture of the lateral tibial rim at the insertion of the fascia lata is unusual and easily overlooked. It is invariably associated with lateral capsular and anterior cruciate ligament tears.[43]

Fractures of the Fibula

Isolated fractures of the proximal fibula are unusual but do occur as oblique or spiral disruptions. These are usually below the insertion of the proximal tibiofibular ligament. A fracture in this location occasionally follows an inversion injury of the ankle (Maisonneuve's fracture). Fracture of the fibula head may accompany a lateral tibial plateau fracture or diastasis of the tibiofibular joint. Assessment of the peroneal nerve should be made.

Fractures of the Patella

Horizontal Fracture

This is the most common patella fracture and usually occurs in the middle zone.

Vertical and Comminuted Fractures

These are uncommon. Displaced fractures require stabilization and, if the patella articular surface cannot be adequately restored, may result in patellectomy.

Flake Fracture

A small osteochondral fragment can be dislodged from the articular surface, especially when there has been traumatic subluxation or dislocation of the patella.

Dislocations of the Knee

Femorotibial Dislocation

Although uncommon, this is a serious injury with popliteal artery and peroneal nerve damage often coexisting. Anterior dislocation is the most common although posterior, lateral, medial, and rotary forms are possible. Any type of dislocation is associated with significant disruption of the capsule and collateral and cruciate ligaments.

Patellofemoral Dislocation

This is the most common dislocation of the knee. Lateral dislocation predominates and is often recurrent. This type of displacement can produce osteochondral (flake) fractures of the patella medial facet or lateral femoral condyle. Predisposing causes in addition to trauma include patella alta, small lateral femoral condyle, shallow patellofemoral grove, genu valgum or recurvatum, lateral insertion of the patella ligament, muscle weakness, and tibial torsion.

Tibiofibular Dislocation

The least common of all knee dislocations, it is also readily overlooked. The usual form is where the fibula head is displaced anteriorly and laterally (anterolateral dislocation).

Stress Fractures

Slowly progressive fractures may occur in normal bone subject to abnormal stress (fatigue or stress fractures) or in abnormal bone (eg, in Paget's disease, osteoporosis, or osteomalacia) subject to normal stress (insufficiency fractures).[44,45] Repetitive activities such as athletic pursuits predispose to these injuries. The knee is the fourth most common site of stress fractures after the spine (pars defects), metatarsals, and the ankle.

Imaging features may be sparse and difficult to identify. Key signs include a subtle fracture line, hazy sclerosis adjacent to the fracture, and periosteal new bone. Bone scan is the most sensitive method available for detection.

Distal Femur

This is an unusual site for stress fractures, although long-distance running, ballet dancing, and marching may precipitate this injury.

Proximal Tibia

This is the most common site for stress fracture at the knee. The fracture is usually found within 5 cm of the articulation and is best seen at the medial cortex of the tibia (Figure 4–26). Predisposing activities include long-distance running, dancing, football, netball, basketball, and marching.

Proximal Fibula

The stress fracture typically lies within 5 cm of the tibiofibular joint and is almost as common as its counterpart in the proximal tibia. Changing from a soft to a hard running surface (runner's fracture) and activities involving repetitive jumping are commonly related activities.[46]

Patella

This is a very rare site but has been reported to involve the superior pole in hurdlers.[45]

Ligamentous Injuries

Imaging of the intraarticular and periarticular knee structures traditionally has been dependent on arthrography. MR imaging increasingly is providing more accurate delineation of these structures and is now the modality of choice in their assessment.

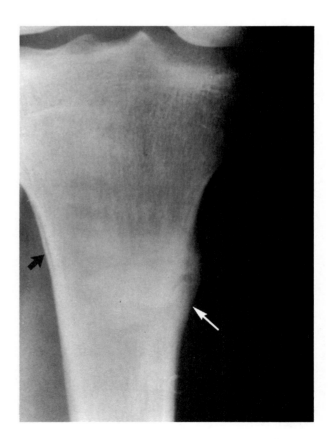

Figure 4–26 Stress fracture of the tibia. Approximately 5 cm medially below the joint, there is a hazy zone of sclerosis and periosteal new bone (arrows). *Comment*: This is the most common site of stress fractures at the knee. In the early stages of the fracture plain films are often normal, but bone scan will clearly isolate the defect.

The only reliable plain film sign of ligamentous injury is calcification at the femoral insertion of the medial collateral ligament some months after injury (Pellegrini-Stieda disease; Figure 4–27). All ligaments are readily seen on MR images as low-signal structures. This is particularly true of the cruciate ligaments, where sensitivity for identifying tears approaches 95%.[12] Ligamentous injury is characterized by abnormal signal (tear or edema), abnormal morphology, or absence of signal (Figure 4–28).

Myositis Ossificans (Myositis Ossificans Traumatica, Heterotopic Ossification, Pseudomalignant Myositis Ossificans)

Clinical Features

Myositis ossificans is a benign, solitary, self-limiting, ossifying soft tissue mass typically occurring within muscle. Trauma is the usual antecedent, although hemorrhage due to a bleeding disorder or anticoagulant therapy and even immobilization may produce similar bone masses.

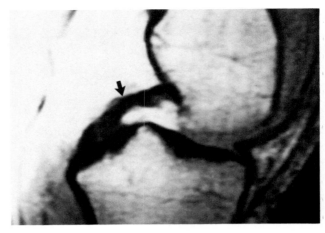

A

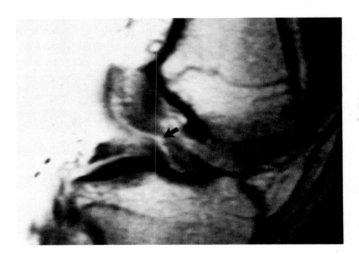

B

Figure 4–28 MR scan of the cruciate ligaments. (**A**) Normal posterior cruciate ligament. The low-signal ligament is seen to be intact and attached to the femur and tibia (arrow). (**B**) Disrupted anterior cruciate ligament. The ligament is almost discontinuous in its midportion as a result of an incomplete rupture (arrow). *Comment*: Disruption of the posterior cruciate ligament is an unusual lesion but can be depicted clearly on MR scan. Tears of the anterior cruciate are similarly well visualized on MR scan, which clearly highlights this modality's application to diagnosing internal derangement of the knee.

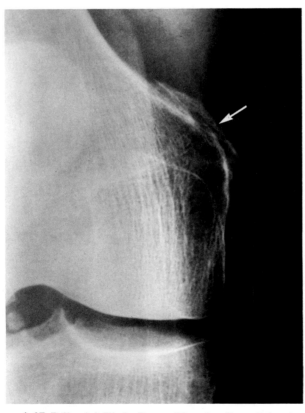

Figure 4–27 Pellegrini-Stieda disease. There is a linear flake of calcification adjacent to the medial epicondyle (arrow). *Comment*: This appearance is due to severe trauma to the insertion of the medial collateral ligament, resulting in transformation of the hematoma to bone. Such a finding may be associated with functional disability of the knee joint. Courtesy of Inger F. Villadsen, DC, Newcastle, Australia.

Blunt trauma to the quadriceps is the most common cause around the knee. Pain, swelling, and bruising occur early. Gradually a localized mass becomes evident that shrinks, hardens, and becomes more palpable. Eventually a hard mass remains with variable degrees of diminished muscle function. Avulsion injury of the medial collateral ligament at its femoral attachment may produce calcification (Pellegrini-Stieda disease), which is a manifestation of the same process.

Imaging Features

Plain radiographs show faint calcification within 2 to 6 weeks after the onset of symptoms. This becomes more definite as externally an undulating cortical border develops by 6 to 8 weeks and shrinks to become mature by 5 to 6 months (Figure 4–29). On CT this rim is evident earlier with lower attenuation internally. MR scan shows edema in the early and intermediate stages with increased signal on T2-weighted images. Throughout the organizing mass there is a heterogeneous signal. Mature lesions are also heterogeneous centrally with a rim of decreased signal.[47]

Meniscal Injuries (Meniscus Tear)

Clinical Features

Meniscal injuries are the most common disorders of the knee joint. They may be traumatic or degenerative in nature. The medial meniscus is injured far more commonly than the lateral meniscus because of its larger length, its reduced mobility, and the frequency of valgus forces. Clinical features are diverse but characteristically show locking, loss of extension, moderate effusion, and articular noises on McMurray's maneuver.

Imaging Features

Traditionally, arthrography has been the mainstay for diagnosis. Arthroscopy has displaced this as both a diagnostic and a therapeutic procedure. Presently MR scan is the noninvasive technique of choice with sensitivity as high as 95%.[12]

Coronal and sagittal images are obtained with a T1-spin echo and narrow windows to demonstrate meniscal detail. Effusion is best seen on T2-weighted images. Tears are identified as abnormal signal within the meniscus, which normally is a homogenous density. Degenerative tears tend to be horizontal, and traumatic disruptions are more vertical[12,48] (Figure 4–30).

The following grades of tears have been described[12]:

- Grade 1: global loss of signal within the meniscus that does not extend to the articular surface; represents degenerative change
- Grade 2: linear loss of signal within the meniscus that does not extend to the surface; also represents degeneration
- Grade 3: loss of signal extending to the articular surface; represents a meniscal tear

MR imaging is especially useful in the evaluation of the postmeniscectomy knee for incompletely excised tears, retained fragments, or other abnormalities. When meniscectomy has been performed, signs of degenerative joint disease are common. Early plain film signs are the development of a ridge of bone from the femoral and tibial margins (Fairbank's sign),

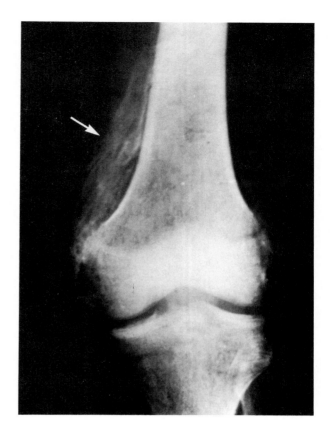

A

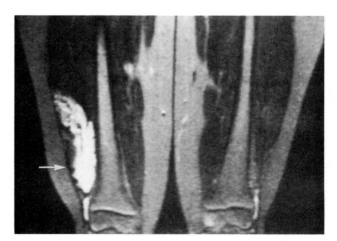

B

Figure 4–29 Myositis ossificans. (**A**) A fine, veil-like opacity is evident over the medial aspect of the distal femur (arrow). Note the mature cortical bone at the periphery of the lesion, which is one of the hallmarks of this process. (**B**) On MR examination the presence of intramuscular hematoma within the vastus lateralis is exquisitely shown (arrow). *Comment:* Hematomas in the first few weeks of their evolution are optimally shown on MR images. It is only in more mature lesions that sufficient calcium is present to allow identification on conventional radiograph.

flattening of the articular surface, and diminished joint space.[25, 49]

Occult traumatic injuries such as a bruised bone are best evaluated by MR scan; there is reduced marrow signal on T1-weighted images and increased signal on T2-weighted images.[12]

Osgood-Schlatter Disease (Traction Apophysitis [Osteochondritis] of the Tibial Tuberosity)

Clinical Features

Osgood-Schlatter disease traditionally implied the pathologic process of avascular necrosis of the tibial tuberosity in the young patient, resulting in fragmentation, pain, and overlying soft tissue swelling. The misnomer and confusing term *osteochondritis* has also been applied.

The disorder is the result of repetitive avulsion forces applied to the tibial tuberosity–patella ligament insertion, where small fragments of cartilage and bone tissue are displaced with a resultant inflammatory response. With time these osteocartilaginous fragments undergo enlargement, the overlying tissues become edematous, and the patella ligament thickens. The clinical expressions of this underlying process are localized swelling and tenderness over the tibial tuberosity, which in chronic cases can be prominent. Up to 25% of cases can be bilateral and in different stages of evolution. Adults can at times reactivate their adolescent syndrome.

Imaging Features

Osgood-Schlatter disease is a clinical diagnosis, not an imaging diagnosis, because plain films can be unremarkable in the presence of significant clinical symptoms. Plain lateral radiographs should be obtained bilaterally, preferably with two exposures (high- and low-kilovolt exposures).[50] For optimal demonstration, 5° of internal rotation of the tibia is required in the lateral projection. Signs include soft tissue swelling, opacified infrapatellar fat, a thickened patella ligament, irregular anterior contour of the tibial tuberosity, and free ossicles (Figure 4–31). The growth plate beneath the tibial tuberosity should not be mistaken as a manifestation of the disease. Occasionally a high-riding patella (patella alta) may be found in association.[50] CT scan will demonstrate bony ossicles and soft tissue signs; bone scans may show focal uptake when the disease is active. MR imaging is especially useful showing edema and soft tissue details.

Sinding-Larsen-Johansson Disease (Patella Apophysitis)

Clinical Features

This is a disease affecting adolescents, most commonly between 10 and 14 years, consisting of tenderness and soft tissue swelling over the lower pole of the patella. It is analogous to Osgood-Schlatter disease in that recurrent trauma causes traction on the patella ligament, precipitating tendinitis, calcifica-

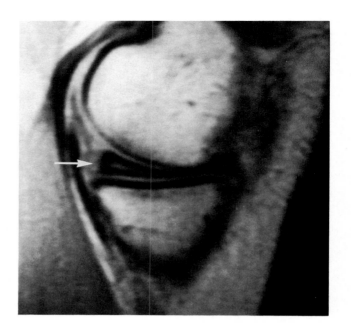

A

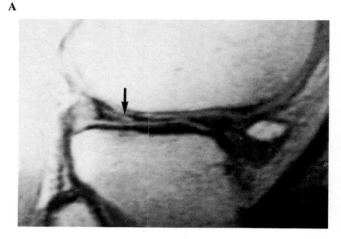

B

Figure 4–30 MR imaging of meniscus tears. (**A**) A horizontal degenerative tear is seen in the posterior horn of the medial meniscus (arrow). (**B**) A vertical traumatic tear can be discerned extending through the posterior aspect of the lateral meniscus (arrow). *Comment*: MR imaging is the modality of choice for the investigation of internal structural derangement. Meniscal tears are readily shown; traumatic tears tend to be vertical, and degenerative defects manifest as horizontal clefts.

tion, or avulsion of bone fragments from the inferior pole of the patella (Figure 4–32).

Imaging Features

On the lateral view, small, separated bony ossicles can be seen distal to the inferior pole of the patella. A soft tissue study may demonstrate soft tissue swelling, thickening of the patella ligament, and effacement of the adjacent infrapatella fat–

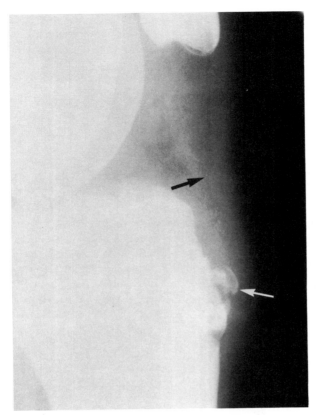

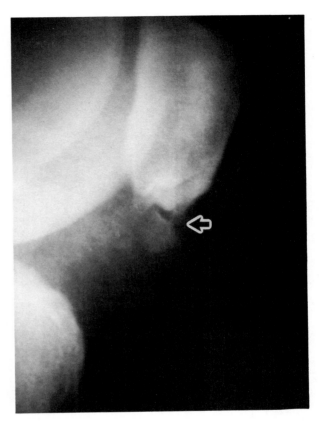

Figure 4–31 Osgood-Schlatter disease. Note the isolated bony ossicles adjacent to the tibial tuberosity (white arrow) and the loss of clear depiction of the infrapatellar fat (Hoffa's fat pad), which indicates edematous infiltration (black arrow). *Comment:* The loss of clear demarcation between Hoffa's fat pad and the patellar ligament is a reliable sign of active inflammation from adjacent traction apophysitis. Courtesy of James R. Brandt, DC, FACO, Coon Rapids, Minnesota.

Figure 4–32 Sinding-Larsen-Johansson disease. Observe the isolated ossicle adjacent to the inferior pole of the patella (arrow), which is irregular. *Comment:* This lesion is analogous to Osgood-Schlatter disease, representing a traction apophysitis of the inferior patellar pole.

patella ligament interface. On resolution, the ossicles may be reincorporated into the patella or remain isolated.

Osteochondritis Dissecans (Transchondral Fracture, König's Disease, Joint Mouse)

Clinical Features

Historically this well-known disorder has been considered to represent a manifestation of a localized subarticular zone of avascular necrosis (osteochondritis). The most likely cause is trauma where there is impaction between the tibial eminences and femoral condyle. As the name suggests, it is a condition of bone and overlying cartilage being dissected away from their attachments. Most defects are discovered between the ages of 10 to 20 years, and there is a male predominance. A broad spectrum of clinical manifestations is found, including pain, effusion, crepitus, and locking; the disorder may even be asymptomatic. Almost one third of cases occur bilaterally.

Imaging Features

The femoral medial condyle is affected in 85% of cases and the lateral condyle in the remaining 15%. Occasionally after dislocation of the patella, a small osteochondral flake may be dislodged from the femoral surface.

The medial condylar lesion characteristically occurs at the lateral margin bordering the intercondylar surface. Lateral condylar lesions involve the weight-bearing surface. Conventional films show a concave, lucent defect (Figure 4–33). This may be obscured on the AP view but can be seen clearly on the AP intercondylar view. The lateral film can often locate the defect on the anterior condylar surface. The sequestered ossicle varies from an oval shape to a linear flake. It may or may not be closely opposed to the site of origin. CT will usually show the defect more completely, although the fragment may not be seen. MR signs around the defect show diminished signal in the subchondral bone and separated fragment. If a zone of high signal is present between the fragment and the femur, this is indicative of stability with firm attachment between the two.[51]

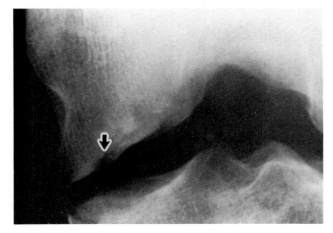

A

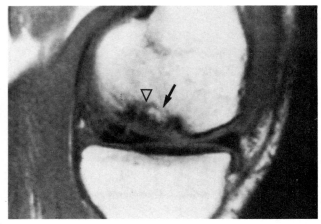

B

Figure 4–33 Osteochondritis dissecans. **(A)** On this tunnel projection the defect and contained fragment can be seen in the characteristic location at the lateral aspect of the medial condyle (arrow). **(B)** On MR scan the crater can be identified as a low-signal (black) zone (arrowhead); the separated fragment is of higher signal intensity (arrow). Careful inspection of the posterior horn of the medial meniscus reveals a horizontal tear. *Comment*: The use of MR imaging in the evaluation of this condition is clearly demonstrated because unsuspected intraarticular lesions can be readily identified. The extent of the underlying osteonecrosis can be seen and the integrity of the hyaline cartilage assessed.

ARTHRITIC DISORDERS

Degenerative Joint Disease (Osteoarthritis, Degenerative Arthritis)

Clinical Features

Degenerative joint disease is the most common form of arthritis to involve the knee. Although the exact triggering mechanism is undefined, the altered biomechanical forces that follow trauma play an integral role. In women there may be a hereditary predisposition, especially in the presence of Heberdeen's nodes of the distal interphalangeal joints. There frequently exists great disparity between the clinical manifesta-

tions and radiographic changes. Common symptoms include pain and stiffness that are worse in the morning and in cold weather but improve with movement. Clinical signs may be few such as crepitus, valgus deformity, bony enlargement, low-grade swelling, and reduced movement.

Imaging Features

The key signs of a degenerative joint are nonuniform loss of joint space, osteophytes, sclerosis, subchondral cysts, subluxation, and occasionally intraarticular loose bodies.

Femorotibial Joint. There is a clear predisposition of early and more marked disease to involve the medial femorotibial joint (Figure 4–34). Nonuniform loss of medial joint space is characteristic. Osteophytes are usually small and inconspicuous until the degeneration becomes severe; this is best seen at the medial tibial and femoral surfaces. Subchondral sclerosis is often mild or virtually absent until advanced disease becomes apparent. Subchondral cysts (geodes) are commonly absent and, if present, tend to be small (less than 5 mm). Tibial geodes are more common than those at the femur and are most

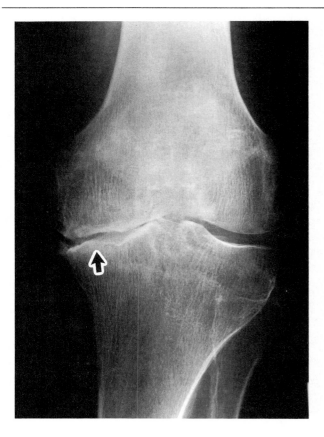

Figure 4–34 Degenerative joint disease of the femorotibial joint. There is characteristic loss of medial joint space (arrow) as well as osteophytes and lateral tibial shift. A few subchondral cysts are apparent beneath the tibial eminences. *Comment*: This asymmetric loss of medial joint space is a good differential feature from rheumatoid arthritis, which tends to narrow both the medial and the lateral joint compartments.

prevalent below the tibial eminences in the posterior tibia. Lateral shift of the femur on the tibia parallels the diminution in the medial joint space. Intraarticular loose bodies are a relatively common association and should be sought on all studies. These will calcify in up to 50% of cases and be visible radiographically as round, sometimes laminated opacities. They should not be confused with the fabella. Occasionally there may be associated chondrocalcinosis. MR scan is particularly useful in depicting degenerative menisci and articular cartilage.

Patellofemoral Joint. Degenerative joint disease at the patellofemoral joint is usually found in combination with disease at the femorotibial joint. Isolated patellofemoral joint disease suggests the presence of pseudogout. The changes are best seen on lateral and tangential views as a loss of joint space, sclerosis, and osteophytes from the poles of the patella (Figure 4–35). An early sign is loss of the lateral patellofemoral joint space. In advanced cases a smooth extrinsic erosion of the anterior femoral surface can be observed. Degenerative ossification on the nonarticular anterior patella surface appears as irregular, vertical, bony spicules separated by lucent zones on the tangential view (patella tooth sign), which is

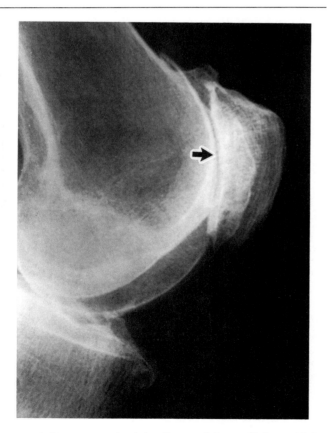

Figure 4–35 Degenerative joint disease of the patellofemoral joint. There is pronounced loss of the patellofemoral joint space (arrow). Some sclerosis and marginal osteophytes can also be seen. *Comment*: Isolated degeneration of the patellofemoral joint space is usually due to pseudogout.

an age-related variant and not a sign of intrinsic articular disease.[52]

Differential Diagnosis

Calcium pyrophosphate dihydrate (CPPD) crystal deposition disease (pseudogout) is the most common and difficult differential possibility. Clinically the manifestations are more acute, inflammatory (hot and swollen), and short lived. Radiographic signs include chondrocalcinosis, synovial calcification, isolated patellofemoral disease, and widespread tricompartmental disease (mediolateral femorotibial and patellofemoral joints).

Chondromalacia Patellae

Clinical Features

Chondromalacia patellae describes the pathologic finding of patellar cartilage degeneration. It is one of the more common causes of knee pain in the adolescent and young adult. Whether cartilage injury in the young patient predisposes to adult patellofemoral arthritis remains controversial. Clinical features consist of a spectrum of presentations ranging from vague to severe anterior knee pain (accentuated by patellofemoral compression), crepitus, and collapse. Protracted knee flexion such as in sitting aggravates the pain (movie sign).

The diagnosis is usually made on clinical grounds and is confirmed with arthroscopy because the imaging features generally lack sensitivity, although the advent of MR imaging has altered this perception.

Imaging Features

Plain film features are unusual, although occasionally irregularity of the patella surface can be identified (Figure 4–36). Arthrography can also demonstrate these features in addition to cartilage fissuring. CT has been generally disappointing, although loss of cartilage and bony irregularity can be depicted. MR scans, both T2-weighted and T1-weighted sequences, exquisitely detail patellar cartilage abnormalities with an accuracy of at least 80% on the basis of either a focal globular or a linear increase in signal.[53]

Rheumatoid Arthritis

Clinical Features

Rheumatoid arthritis is a common inflammatory disorder of synovial joints and connective tissue. The time of onset is usually between 20 and 60 years of age, with a peak incidence between 40 and 50 years. Women younger than 40 years are three times more frequently involved than men of the same age; after 40 there is an equal sex distribution.

Signs and symptoms are variable. The most obvious feature is polyarticular inflammatory joint disease, often of the peripheral joints of the hands and feet. Systemic features can in-

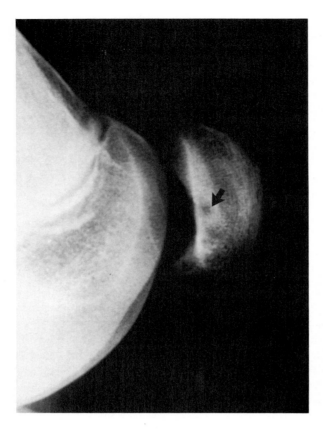

Figure 4–36 Chondromalacia patellae. Discrete cystic lucencies are present at the articular surface of the patella (arrow). Note the femoral growth plate in this 14-year-old girl. *Comment*: Most plain film studies of chondromalacia patellae are unrewarding, although occasionally these changes may be evident. MR scan is the imaging method of choice to show cartilaginous defects.

clude fever, weight loss, fatigue, muscle soreness, and anemia. Up to 70% of patients have a positive rheumatoid arthritis latex test. The erythrocyte sedimentation rate is usually elevated, and antinuclear antibody is often positive. Involvement of the knee is common and may occur early or late in the disease process. Early there is evidence of effusion, warmth, and stiffness. Baker's cysts are common and can be large. Later muscle atrophy of the quadriceps can be marked, and rheumatoid nodules occasionally will occur in the quadriceps tendon.

Imaging Features

Evidence of effusion is seen in the suprapatellar pouch. Osteoporosis, initially juxtaarticular and later more generalized, can be seen. The key is uniform loss of joint space in the medial and lateral femorotibial joint (bicompartmental disease) and occasionally in the patellofemoral joint (tricompartmental disease; Figure 4–37). Small marginal ero-

sions are occasionally seen at the proximal tibia. Large subchondral cystic lesions can occur, particularly in the tibia. Infrequently a solid or a single laminated periosteal response occurs in the distal femur. Varus and valgus deformities may supervene. Nuclear bone scan will show increased uptake on both sides of the joint.

Pseudogout (CPPD Crystal Deposition Disease, Chondrocalcinosis)

Clinical Features

Pseudogout is a crystal-induced articular disorder that has marked similarities to the clinical presentation of gout, from which the term *pseudogout* derives. Rather than monourate crystals of gout within synovial fluid, needle-shaped, birefringent calcium pyrophosphate dihydrate (CPPD) crystals are found. CPPD crystals are deposited into intraarticular chondrocyte lacunae and subsequently are released coincident with chondrocyte death, inciting episodic inflammatory synovitis.

Three forms of presentation occur: acute, chronic, and asymptomatic. In the acute form (20% of cases), the joint is warm, swollen, and tender; these symptoms last for 1 to 7 days. The chronic form (60% of cases) is most common and presents with stiffness, swelling, and crepitus; it is indistin-

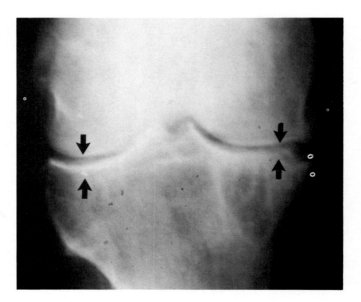

Figure 4–37 Rheumatoid arthritis. There is symmetric loss of both the medial and the lateral joint spaces (arrows). Large subchondral cysts are evident in the tibia; these are uncommon in rheumatoid knee. *Comment*: Such uniform loss of joint space is a hallmark of rheumatoid arthritis; selective compartmental disease is more typical of degenerative joint disease.

guishable from degenerative joint disease. Acute episodes are often superimposed. In the asymptomatic form (20% of cases), there is radiographic evidence only of chondrocalcinosis.

Imaging Features

Pseudogout of the knee can be found in two separate or superimposed forms: chondrocalcinosis and pyrophosphate arthropathy.

Chondrocalcinosis. This may be identified within menisci and hyaline cartilage. Meniscal chondrocalcinosis is readily identified by the triangular shape of the calcification and an often dense lateral meniscus (Figure 4–38). Hyaline chondrocalcinosis manifests as fine, punctate calcifications oriented in a linear pattern paralleling the articular surface. Additional calcification is sometimes seen within the joint capsule, synovial lining, and periarticular ligaments and tendons.

Confirmation of chondrocalcinosis can be made with radiographs of the contralateral knee, wrists (ulnar compartment triangular cartilage), and symphysis pubis. Other causes for chondrocalcinosis include the "three C's": *cation disease* (calcium, hyperparathyroidism; iron, hemochromatosis; and copper, Wilson's disease); *crystal disease* (CPPD, pseudogout; monourate, gout; and homogentisic acid, ochronosis); and *cartilage degeneration* (degenerative joint disease, diabetes, and idiopathic).

Pyrophosphate arthropathy. This is characterized by two features: advanced degenerative changes and an unusual dis-

tribution. Prominent degenerative features are sclerosis, cysts, loose bodies, osteophytes, loss of joint space, and occasionally articular destruction simulating neuropathic arthropathy. Usually there is involvement of the medial femorotibial joint space; this is followed by the patellofemoral compartment and, last, by the lateral femorotibial compartment. Isolated patellofemoral degenerative joint disease should suggest CPPD as the underlying cause.

Synoviochondrometaplasia (Osteochondromatosis, Loose Bodies, Joint Mouse)

Clinical Features

Intraarticular loose bodies may form as a result of osteochondritis dissecans, cartilage fragmentation, or, more commonly, benign synovial metaplasia (which forms multiple cartilaginous foci). It is a disorder found at all ages but usually presents in the 30- to 50-year age group and is more common in men (almost three times more common). The most frequent site is the knee; this is followed by the elbows, ankles, and shoulders.

Clinical manifestations are mild and chronic with pain, effusion, and crepitus. Intermittent joint locking signifies an intraarticular lesion as the loose bodies migrate into the articular contact zone. Once removed, they are prone to recurrence. There is no association with malignant transformation.

Imaging Features

Up to 80% of these cartilaginous foci develop calcification and even ossification to become visible on plain film studies. They may be single or multiple. Each loose body varies in size from 1 to 20 mm; they are round to ovoid and frequently laminated. They can be located anywhere in the suprapatellar pouch or popliteal fossa; they may even occur within a Baker's cyst down into the calf (Figure 4–39).

The fabella should not be confused with synoviochondrometaplasia, which lies in the posterolateral compartment behind the lateral femoral condyle.

Calcific Prepatellar Bursitis (Housemaid's Knee)

Clinical Features

Repetitive trauma to the tissues below the patella may result in chronic inflammation of the prepatellar bursa, the superficial pretibial bursa, and other adventitious bursae along the patella ligament.[25] This results in a painful soft tissue swelling above the tibial tuberosity. Recurrent episodes may result in a calcareous bursal deposit, which renders it hard and nodular on palpation.

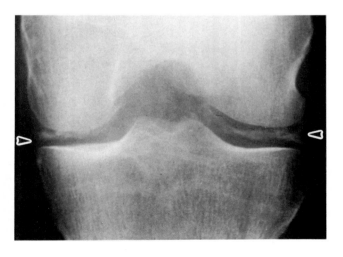

Figure 4–38 Pseudogout. There is marked calcification of both the medial and the lateral menisci (arrowheads). This is designated chondrocalcinosis. *Comment*: This is one manifestation of pseudogout; the other is a destructive and degenerative arthropathy. There are also other causes of chondrocalcinosis (the three C's; see text).

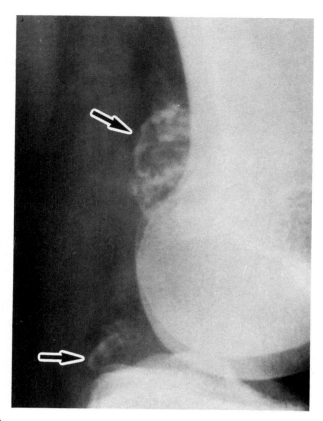

A

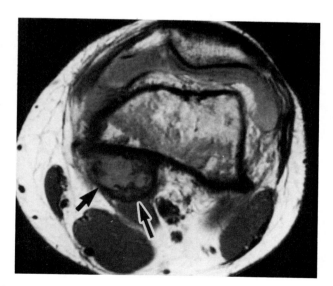

B

Figure 4–39 Synoviochondrometaplasia. (**A**) There are multiple calcified cartilaginous loose bodies at the posterior aspect of the femur and its articulation (arrows). (**B**) On T1-weighted MR scan the posterior femoral loose body is clearly depicted (arrows). *Comment*: Approximately 80% of these lesions will have calcium present, which will allow identification on plain film study.

Imaging Features

On the lateral film round, irregular calcifications can be seen anterior to the patellar ligament (Figure 4–40). Notably, they are not intraarticular. If loose bodies are seen within the joint, they are an unrelated process.

Hypertrophic Osteoarthropathy (Hypertrophic Pulmonary Osteoarthropathy, Marie-Bamberger Syndrome)

Clinical Features

This is an uncommon manifestation of, most commonly, an intrathoracic neoplasm. The disorder is a triad of digital clubbing, symmetric peripheral arthritis, and long bone periostitis. The arthritis is nonspecific with swelling and warmth of the joint, most commonly the knees, ankles, elbows, and wrists. Periostitis manifests as painful legs and forearms, especially on firm pressure.

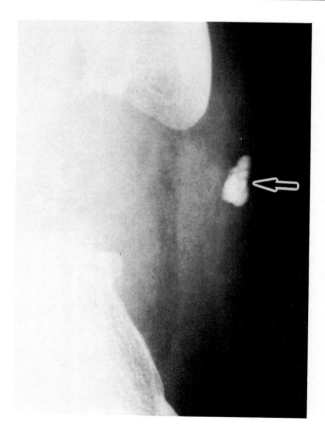

Figure 4–40 Prepatellar bursitis (housemaid's knee). In the chronic form, dense calcifications can occur (arrow). *Comment*: Prepatellar bursitis is a common sequela to prolonged kneeling on hard surfaces, as in carrying out domestic chores, riding a surfboard, or laying carpet.

Imaging Features

The most apparent and consistent radiographic sign is long bone periostitis. At the knee this is evident in the femur, tibia, and fibula as a single laminated or solid periosteal response. This is usually bilateral and restricted to the diaphysis and metaphysis (Figure 4–41). Effusion may be evident in the suprapatellar pouch.

Meniscal Cyst (Ganglion Cyst)

Clinical Features

These most commonly involve the lateral meniscus, which itself is invariably abnormal. They present as a firm swelling at the joint line. Recurrence is common unless the associated meniscal tear is excised. The lesion represents synovial fluid

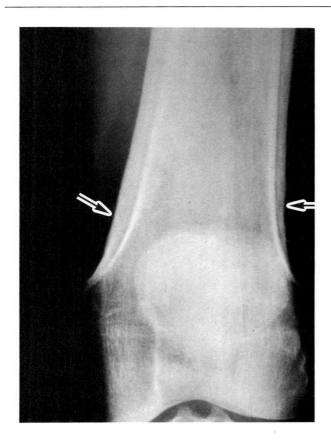

Figure 4–41 Hypertrophic osteoarthropathy. Note the pronounced solid periosteal response on both the medial and the lateral cortices of the distal femur (arrows). The same findings were present on the opposite femur, tibia, and fibula in this patient. *Comment*: This finding of bilateral and symmetric long bone periostitis is usually associated with carcinoma of the lung. It does not represent metastatic disease but is related to reflex altered blood flow. A triad of findings can be present: clubbing of the digits, joint pain, and long bone periostitis.

being forced through a horizontal tear in the meniscus that extends to the meniscocapsular margin.

Imaging Features

MR scan is diagnostic with low signal intensity on T1-weighted images and high signal intensity on T2-weighted images.[12] Its margins are well demarcated, and the communicating meniscal tear may be identified (Figure 4–42).

NEOPLASMS

The knee is a common site for bone tumors because of its high metabolic rate and vascularity. The most common primary malignant bone tumors are multiple myeloma, osteosarcoma, and chondrosarcoma. Secondary (metastatic) tumors are uncommon. Benign tumors occur at the knee much more frequently than malignant tumors. Of the benign tumors osteochondroma is the most common tumor of the knee. Other common benign lesions include nonossifying fibroma, aneurysmal bone cyst, giant cell tumor, and osteoid osteoma.

Osteosarcoma

Clinical Features

Osteosarcoma is the second most common primary bone tumor after multiple myeloma. In the adolescent to young adult stage (10 to 25 years), however, it is the most common. Males are affected almost twice as often as females. Pain and swelling that fail to resolve with conservative measures is the most common presentation. The tumor is often fortuitously when radiographs are obtained. Virtually 60% of all

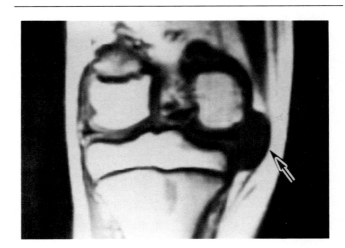

Figure 4–42 Meniscal cyst. On MR scan the cyst is clearly delineated abutting the adjacent torn lateral meniscus (arrow). *Comment*: Meniscal cysts are far more common on the lateral joint line. They are invariably associated with a tear in the ipsilateral meniscus, which allows for the extravasation of synovial fluid.

osteosarcomas occur at the knee, 40% in the distal femur alone.[54] This makes osteosarcoma the most common malignancy to be found at the knee. Survival is unpredictable as a result of metastatic disease, although the poor prognosis of previous decades has been somewhat mitigated. Notably, osteosarcoma and Ewing's sarcoma are the only primary bone tumors to metastasize to other bones.

Imaging Features

Osteosarcoma has a spectrum of presentations, although 90% of lesions are greater than 5 cm, metaphyseal, and sclerotic; disrupt the cortex; and exhibit a spiculated (hair-on-end) or laminated (onion-skin) periosteal response, Codman's triangles, and produce a dense soft tissue mass (cumulus cloud appearance) (Figure 4–43). Approximately 10% are diaphyseal with epiphyseal regions rare. Purely osteolytic presentations are uncommon.

Isotopic bone scan demonstrates strong isotopic uptake and is useful in detecting other bone-forming metastatic deposits. CT assists in delineating the plain film changes, especially the soft tissue mass, which is critical in making the diagnosis. MR scan also is useful in this regard and can define the extent of

bone marrow involvement (to assist in surgical planning) as well as response to chemotherapy.

Chondrosarcoma

Clinical Features

Chondrosarcoma is the third most common primary malignant bone tumor after multiple myeloma and osteosarcoma. It makes up 10% of primary malignant bone tumors, with 50% involving the pelvis and upper femur. Approximately 7% involve the knee region.[54] They may arise as primary tumors or be secondary to osteochondroma, enchondroma, Paget's disease, fibrous dysplasia, or irradiation. They most commonly occur in the 40- to 60-year age group and affect men twice as much as women. Pain and swelling can be mild; therefore, there may be extensive tumor by the time it is discovered.

Imaging Features

Lesions may be predominantly within the bone (central) or near its surface (peripheral). Central chondrosarcomas are largely lytic, geographic-type lesions that may disrupt the cortex. Endosteal scalloping and, in up to two thirds of cases,

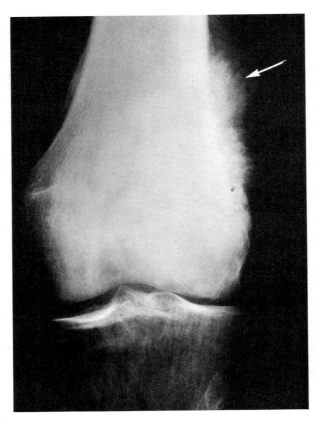

A

Figure 4–43 Osteosarcoma. **(A)** The increased density and periosteal response (arrow) are virtually diagnostic.

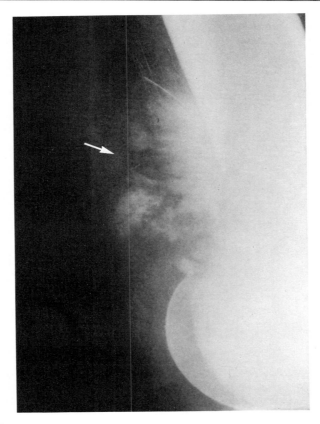

B

Figure 4–43 (B) On the lateral view the spiculated (sunburst) nature of the periosteal response is clearly demonstrated (arrow).

matrix calcification (rings and arcs or popcorn sign) are characteristic. A large soft tissue mass and periosteal new bone are also common. Peripheral chondrosarcomas tend to exhibit less bone change but larger soft tissue mass.

Synovial Sarcoma (Synovioma)

Clinical Features

Synovioma is a rare malignant tumor arising from synovium of joint capsules, bursae, or tendon sheaths. Approximately 50% occur in the vicinity of the knee.[54] Most occur between 20 to 40 years of age and can be rapidly fatal. Pain, tenderness, and a lump that does not enlarge noticeably are characteristic. Rapid growth and metastasis can occur at any time, however.

Imaging Features

A soft tissue mass that is often spheric and around 7 cm in diameter is a consistent feature (Figure 4–44). More than 30% demonstrate fine flecks or linear bands of calcification, which are more obvious on CT examination. Bone involvement is uncommon, although osteoporosis can be seen.

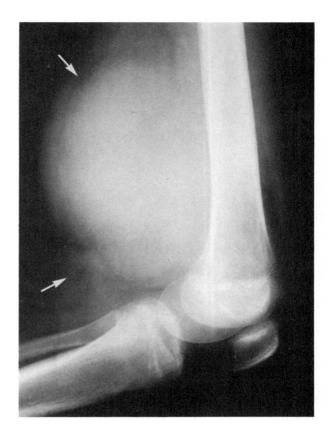

Figure 4–44 Synovial sarcoma. A large soft tissue mass is evident in the posterior thigh (arrows). *Comment*: Synovioma is a rare malignant tumor, although at least 50% occur at the knee. A soft tissue mass is often the only manifestation, although around 30% may calcify.

Ewing's Sarcoma (Malignant Endothelioma)

Clinical Features

This is a rare malignant bone tumor primarily occurring in the second decade of life with a peak age of 15 years. Boys are affected twice as commonly as girls. There is a predilection for the long bone diaphyses, with 20% arising in the femur, 10% in the tibia, and 5% in the fibula.[54] Pain is the usual first symptom; it gradually worsens and is followed by a soft tissue mass. Systemic features of intermittent fever, anemia, and leukocytosis initially confuse the clinical picture with that of osteomyelitis, which often cannot be excluded radiologically.

Imaging Features

Great variation in appearance occurs. The most characteristic appearance is a diaphyseal moth-eaten destruction (cracked ice appearance) surrounded by a laminated periosteal response (Figure 4–45). Some lesions with a soft tissue mass cause an extrinsic destruction of the periosteal new bone and cortex,

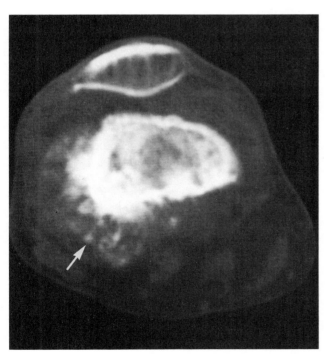

C

Figure 4–43 (C) CT examination with a bone window shows bone involvement as well as periosteal and sarcomatous new bone formation (arrow). *Comment*: Osteosarcoma is the most common malignant tumor of the knee, and the knee is the most frequent site of occurrence of this tumor. The imaging features demonstrated are characteristic in the vast majority of osteosarcomas.

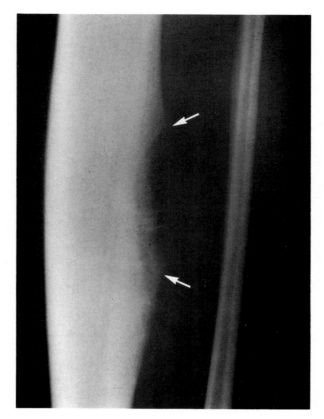

Figure 4–45 Ewing's sarcoma. Along the lateral border of the tibia, note the triangular regions of periosteal response bordering the lesion (Codman's triangles; arrows). Within the lesion, a few scattered vertical periosteal spicules of bone are also evident. Note the characteristic but uncommon scalloped appearance (saucerization). *Comment*: Ewing's sarcoma is usually a diaphyseal lesion of bone. It tends to be centric with diffuse, moth-eaten destruction and is surrounded by a laminated periosteal collar.

creating an externally concave defect (saucerization). MR and CT scans assist in defining the soft tissue mass and bony changes.

Metastatic Carcinoma

Clinical Features

Bony secondaries demonstrate a wide spectrum of presentations from asymptomatic to severely debilitating. Night pain that progressively worsens is a key feature. Pathologic fracture may be an acute presentation. In general, skeletal metastasis is an axial phenomenon, being confined to the spine, pelvis, skull, and ribs. Less frequently the proximal humerus and femurs may be involved. Metastasis is considered rare below the elbow and knee and accounts for less than 1.5% of skeletal secondaries.[54] The most common cause of these limb metastases in more than 90% of cases is carcinoma of the

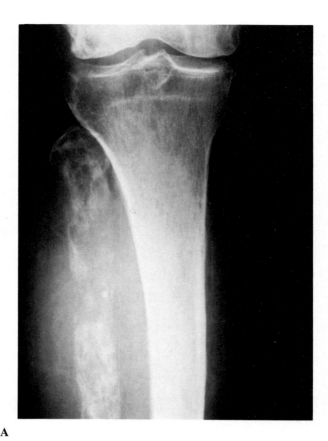

A

Figure 4–46 Metastatic carcinoma. (**A**) Osteolytic form (breast primary). Observe the grossly destructive lesion within the fibula. The lesion has also disrupted the cortex.

lung. Other occasional causes include tumors of the prostate, breast, kidney, and thyroid and melanoma.

Imaging Features

Most lesions are osteolytic with little to no periosteal response. Expansile blow-out and soap bubble metastases are associated with renal and thyroid tumors. Osteoblastic lesions can be focal or diffuse (Figure 4–46).

Osteochondroma (Exostosis)

Clinical Features

An osteochondroma is a benign developmental defect that follows a lateral herniation of an epiphyseal plate. It is the most common tumor of the entire skeleton, with at least 50% being found at the knee (femur, 35%; tibia, 15%).[54] Boys are afflicted slightly more commonly than girls. Histologically the exostosis comprises normal mature bone covered with hyaline cartilage, which is identical to an epiphyseal plate. Growth of an osteochondroma therefore ceases once skeletal maturity is reached. Many lesions are found incidentally on

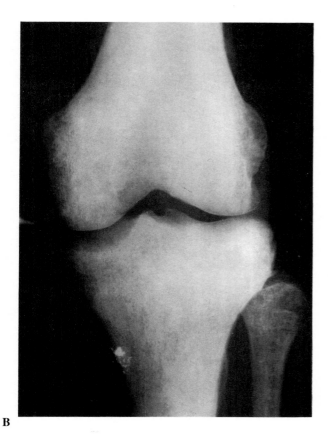

B

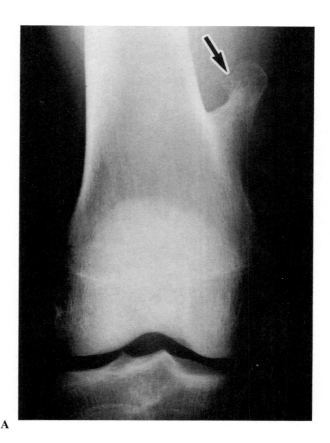

A

Figure 4–46 (B) Osteoblastic form (prostate primary). There is diffuse sclerosis of all bones. This type of presentation will usually have all bones similarly sclerotic. *Comment*: Metastatic carcinoma is rare below the knee. The common primary sites to metastasize in this area are lung, prostate, breast, kidney, and thyroid; melanoma also metastasizes below the knee.

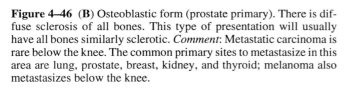

radiographic examination. A common presentation is a painless hard mass near a joint. Less often there may be joint restriction, acute fracture of the stalk, neurovascular compression syndromes, and even popliteal aneurysm. Pain over an osteochondroma may be due to an inflamed overlying adventitious bursa or adjacent tissue. Less than 1% of exostoses may undergo malignant transformation, which is marked clinically by increasing size at a known site of exostosis.

A hereditary form (hereditary multiple exostosis) exists that is male dominant, involves all skeletal growth plates, and may be complicated by malignant transformation in at least 10% of cases.

Imaging Features

These are metaphyseal lesions and have two conformations: pedunculated and sessile.

Pedunculated Osteochondroma. This is the most common variety. It exhibits a bone stalk of variable length that is oriented away from the joint (Figure 4–47). The cap of the lesion

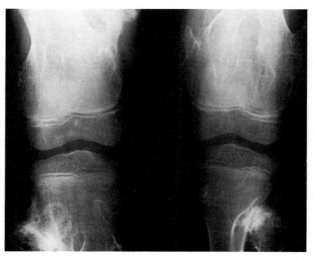

B

Figure 4–47 Osteochondroma, pedunculated form. **(A)** Solitary form. There is a prominent bony exostosis extending off the lateral femur (arrow). Note the thin cortex of the cap, whose resemblance to malignant change can be misleading. **(B)** Multiple form. Numerous osteochondromas can be seen originating from all bones. They remain consistent in their orientation away from the nearest joint. *Comment*: Osteochondroma has the dual distinction of being the most common benign tumor of the entire skeleton and the most common tumor of the knee. The lesions are invariably oriented away from the nearest joint. Courtesy of Inger F. Villadsen, DC, Newcastle, Australia.

is often irregular, seems to lack cortex and may be calcified to a variable extent. When the exostosis is seen en face, there is an ovoid radiolucency corresponding to the origin of the stalk.

Sessile Osteochondroma. The major morphologic feature is the broad base at the point of origin. This may simulate an expansile neoplasm such as an aneurysmal bone cyst because the cortex is thin and the internal trabecular matrix is sparse. Some calcification may be evident in the cap. Isotopic bone scan often demonstrates activity in the cap, especially in skeletally immature individuals.

Nonossifying Fibroma (Fibroxanthoma, Nonosteogenic Fibroma, Fibrous Cortical Defect, Caffey's Defect)

Clinical Features

These lesions are extremely common in the first two decades of life, with up to 40% of normal children probably having one or more such defects.[55] Up to 95% are discovered in individuals younger than 20 years. *Fibrous cortical defect* (Caffey's defect) is the term applied to the same lesion when found in patients younger than 8 years. At least 75% occur at the knee, most often the distal femur. The majority are asymptomatic lesions discovered incidentally on radiographs obtained for another reason, especially trauma. Occasionally, if large, they may precipitate pathologic fracture or insufficiency fractures. They do not undergo malignant transformation. The natural history of most defects is involution and healing. Large lesions in critical sites may require surgical curettage and packing. Numerous nonossifying fibromas have been observed to coexist with neurofibromatosis.

Imaging Features

The characteristic appearance of nonossifying fibroma is an elongated, tapered (flame-shaped) lesion eccentrically placed in a long bone metaphysis (Figure 4–48). It occasionally can extend into the diaphysis. Other diagnostic features include a scalloped sclerotic margin, cortical thinning, and slight expansion. Evidence of resolution is diminishing size and the appearance of sclerotic foci that enlarge and coalesce, progressively filling in the lesion. These are usually active on isotopic bone scan.

Aneurysmal Bone Cyst

Clinical Features

This is an expansile lesion that is the only bone tumor to be named by its radiographic appearance (it looks like an arterial

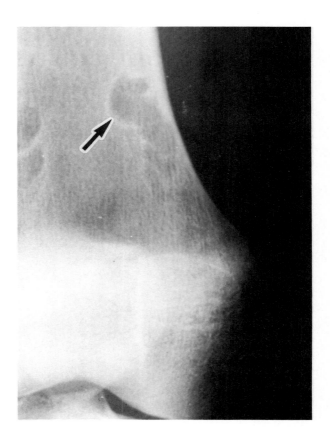

Figure 4–48 Nonossifying fibroma. There is an eccentric, scalloped bony defect in the femoral metaphysis (arrow). *Comment*: Nonossifying fibromas are extremely common benign bone lesions in the developing skeleton and occur most frequently close to the knee joint. As a rule, they do not cause clinical symptoms but when large may predispose to pathologic fracture.

aneurysm) rather than on the basis of histology. Aneurysmal bone cysts usually occur within the first three decades of life with equal sex distribution. Trauma appears to be a precipitant in a number of cases. The distal femur and proximal tibia are the most common sites.[56] Increasing pain over a relatively short period is the main form of presentation.

Imaging Features

The most conspicuous feature is a metaphyseal lesion that is expansile, lightly septated, and contained within a thin, peripheral, calcified (eggshell) rim (Figure 4–49). In the fibula it may be purely centrically located; in the larger femur and tibia eccentricity is the rule. At the base of the lesion is a reactive buttress (Codman's triangle), which signifies its active expansile nature. On isotope study there is active uptake at the

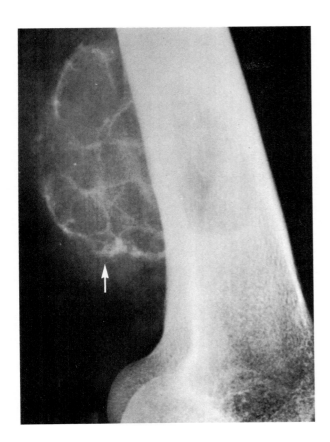

Figure 4–49 Aneurysmal bone cyst. At the posterior aspect of the distal femur, an expansile septated tumor is clearly seen (arrow). Observe in particular the thin peripheral rim. *Comment*: These tumors grow quickly and cause moderate to severe pain.

tumor site. CT delineates the morphology with greater resolution, especially the thin rim, which may confirm the diagnosis and help exclude a malignant tumor. MR imaging allows clear depiction of its internal vascularity, occasional fluid levels and septation with clarification of the relationship to adjacent structures, which is useful in surgical planning.

Giant Cell Tumor (Osteoclastoma)

Clinical Features

This tumor carries the distinction of being a quasi-malignant tumor: 80% are benign, and 20% are malignant. Benign giant cell tumor (GCT) can also transform into a malignant form, generally in the first 5 years after discovery. Most GCTs arise between the ages of 20 and 40 years. Men exhibit a higher incidence of malignant forms and women of the benign forms. Up to 60% of GCTs occur at the knee, most commonly

the distal femur and then the tibia, the fibula, and, rarely, the patella.[54] Presentation is due to low-grade persistent pain or pathologic fracture.

Imaging Features

The hallmark of the tumor is its involvement of both the metaphysis and the epiphysis, extending to the subarticular plate. In addition, it tends to lie slightly eccentrically and causes scalloping and thinning of the cortex externally, while internally discrete septa are clearly visible (Figure 4–50). Isotope studies demonstrate increased uptake. CT and MR scans define the morphology in greater detail.

The radiographic appearance is inconsistent with the tumor being histologically benign or malignant.

Pigmented Villonodular Synovitis (Benign Synovioma)

Clinical Features

Pigmented villonodular synovitis is a benign disorder with diffuse or localized hyperplasia of the synovial villi and hemosiderin deposition. The most common site is the knee.[54] Young adults are usually involved, presenting with swelling but little pain. Aspiration often fails to reduce the effusion, and the aspirate is bloodstained and high in cholesterol content.

Imaging Features

Plain film findings are nonspecific and include soft tissue swelling that may be dense and lobulated, normal joint space, and, rarely, extrinsic bone erosion (Figure 4–51). On MR scan the lobulated intraarticular mass can be defined. On T1-weighted images areas of fat and hemorrhage will be of high signal intensity; on T2-weighted images there is decreased signal due to hemosiderin and chronic synovial proliferation. On CT scan the high iron content results in high attenuation numbers of the mass.

VASCULAR DISORDERS

Clinical Features

Vascular disorders around the knee are not uncommon. They may involve the arteries or veins. Arterial disorders may include atherosclerosis, aneurysms, and thrombosis. Venous problems mostly manifest as thrombophlebitis. Arterial clinical signs include claudication and the "five P's" of arterial obstruction: reduced distal pulses, pallor, a painfully cold extremity, paresthesia, and paralysis. Aneurysms of the popliteal artery produce a pulsatile mass in the popliteal fossa; these are often bilateral and usually occur in concert with abdominal aortic aneurysm.[57] Thrombophlebitis is characterized by calf pain that is exacerbated by ankle dorsiflexion (Homans' sign) and edema below the thrombus.

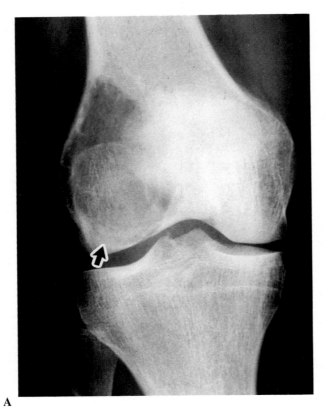

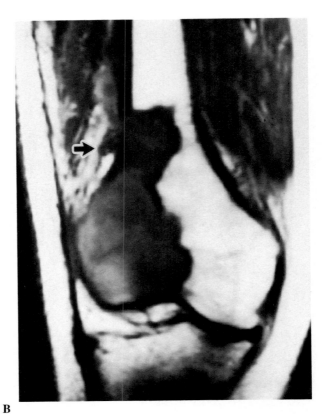

A B

Figure 4–50 Giant cell tumor (GCT). (**A**) Plain film. Within the lateral femoral condyle is a geographic lesion that extends into the subarticular region (arrow). (**B**) MR image. On this T1-weighted image the extent of the tumor can be appreciated; the destruction of the cortex laterally (arrow) is not visible on the plain film study. *Comment:* GCTs can be malignant despite their benign appearance on plain films. MR imaging has the ability to depict clearly a soft tissue mass consistent with a malignant form, as shown in this case.

Imaging Features

Plain films are largely unhelpful. Evidence of atheroma can be seen with calcification of the subintimal plaques. Calcification of the vascular media is common in diabetes and can be seen as sequential, closely opposed rings. Aneurysms occasionally exhibit peripheral calcification, which allows their identification (Figure 4–52). Ultrasound and angiography are essential for depiction of most vascular lesions.

Spontaneous Osteonecrosis of the Knee (SONK)

Clinical Features

SONK is a disorder of the weight-bearing position of the femoral condyle. It has been regarded incorrectly as the adult equivalent of adolescent osteochondritis dissecans. SONK occurs in the population older than 50 years and affects women more commonly than men.[58] The medial condyle is involved in at least 85% of cases; of the remainder, the lateral condyle is involved in 10% and the tibial condyles in 5%. SONK is rarely

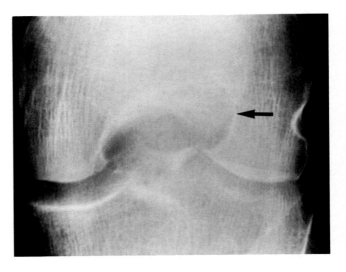

Figure 4–51 Pigmented villonodular synovitis. There is expansion of the intercondylar notch laterally (arrow). No other abnormalities are present. *Comment:* Plain film findings in this lesion are uncommon because the joint capsule is distensible and inhibits extrinsic bone erosion.

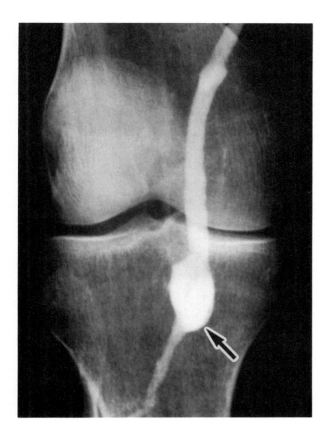

Figure 4–52 Popliteal aneurysm. On the angiogram, note the saccular expansion of the popliteal artery (arrow). *Comment*: Popliteal aneurysms usually coexist bilaterally and frequently are associated with abdominal aortic aneurysms.

bilateral.[59] A history of sudden and severe pain without significant trauma both with exercise and at rest is typical. Physical signs include tenderness of the knee joint, especially over the involved condyle, and effusion. Bone collapse, varus deformity, and secondary degenerative changes can complicate the disease. Recorded causes of SONK include corticosteroids, osteopenia, pancreatitis, lupus erythematosus, occlusive vascular disease, sickle cell anemia, caisson disease, Gaucher's disease, and alcoholism. Pathologically there is osteonecrosis, which may be due to primary vascular obstruction or a fracture in osteopenic bone that disturbs its vascularity distally.

Small lesions with minimal collapse can heal and result in minimal flattening of the condylar surface. More frequently, where the defect involves more than 50% of the condyle, collapse of the articular surface ensues and rapidly progresses to severe secondary degenerative arthritis.[58]

Imaging Features

Plain film changes may take weeks to months to appear, although as early as 5 weeks after the first symptoms diagnostic features can occur.[59]

The major findings include flattening of the articular surface, subchondral sclerosis, subchondral fracture, and the formation of a pitlike radiolucent defect. Less commonly, iso-

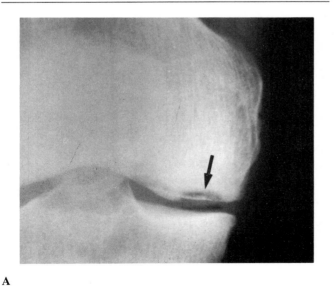

A

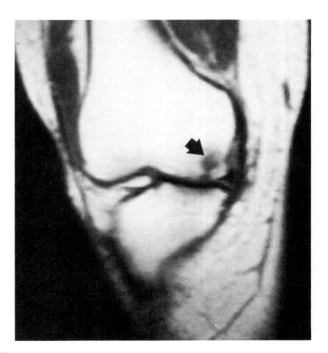

B

Figure 4–53 Spontaneous Osteonecrosis of the Knee (SONK). (**A**) Plain film. On the weight-bearing surface of the medial femoral condyle, there is a linear lucency that has separated a flake of articular bone (arrow). (**B**) MR scan. There is localized decreased signal intensity extending into the medial femoral condyle (arrow). *Comment:* It can be a rapidly destructive condition and must be recognized early to avoid severe joint dysfunction.

lated bone fragments can be seen (Figure 4–53). Periosteal new bone occasionally is present at the distal femur. Bone scan is confirmatory, with intense radionuclide uptake in the involved condyle.

The application of CT and MR scans is to define more accurately the anatomic pathology. On MR scan in the early phases, there is decreased signal on T1-weighted images that may be present when all other studies, including bone scan, are normal. Persistence of low intensity on T2-weighted images (black on black) is a useful feature differentiating SONK from tumor and infection.[59]

Bone Infarct (Localized Bone Death)

Clinical Features

A wide spectrum of presentations occurs, with no specific cluster of symptoms being diagnostic. Many bone infarcts are found incidentally on radiographs, whereas others cause nonspecific knee pain. Causes include pancreatitis, lupus erythematosus, alcoholism, caisson disease, Gaucher's disease, sickle cell anemia, and vascular occlusive disease. For many bone infarcts, the cause remains undetermined. The distal femur and proximal tibia are common sites of involvement.

Imaging Features

In the early stages of infarction, plain films may be normal or may demonstrate a subtle admixture of mottled rarefaction and sclerosis within the medullary cavity of the diametaphyseal region (Figure 4–54). MR scan at this stage shows intermediate signal intensity on T1-weighted images and high signal on T2-weighted images internally; these areas are delineated peripherally by a thin, low-signal band. Mature bone infarcts exhibit a densely calcified, serpiginous border surrounding a central lucent zone. These older infarcts are of low signal on T1- and T2-weighted images.[60]

INFECTIONS

Presentation of bone and joint infections depends on the underlying organism, host defense, and preexisting abnormalities. The most common organism in at least 90% of cases is *Staphylococcus aureus*. Four patterns of skeletal infection are evident: acute osteomyelitis, chronic osteomyelitis, Brodie's abscess, and septic arthritis.

Acute Osteomyelitis (Bone Infection, Skeletal Sepsis)

Clinical Features

The tibia is the most common bone affected by osteomyelitis; it is followed by the femur. Pain, swelling, malaise, and fever are the most striking clinical signs.

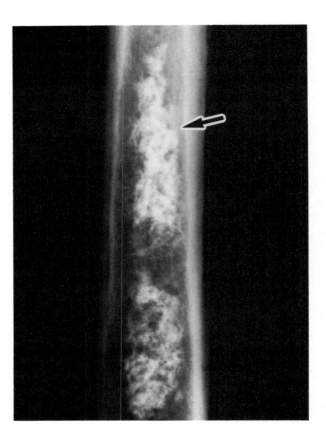

Figure 4–54 Bone infarct. Observe the diffuse and irregular calcification within the medullary cavity (arrow). *Comment*: These are relatively common, asymptomatic bone lesions and occur most frequently within the femur and tibia, often close to the knee.

Imaging Features

It may take a minimum of 10 days (radiographic latent period) before plain film changes become visible. These consist of moth-eaten destruction, isolated necrotic bone fragments (sequestra), and, if periosteal new bone is proliferative, formation of an involucrum (Figure 4–55). Fat planes tend to be obliterated. Gallium-67 bone scans are especially useful in early-stage depiction of these changes, although ^{99m}Tc scans will also show increased uptake at the infective site.[61] The metaphysis is the most common site for involvement. When there is spread into the joint from a metaphyseal focus, this is designated a Tom Smith arthritis.[62]

Chronic Osteomyelitis (Garré's Sclerosing Osteomyelitis)

Clinical Features

Failure of therapy or body defense mechanisms to obliterate the organism can result in an ongoing and unresolved osteomyelitis. This not uncommonly follows fractures of the tibia or femur. Low-grade pain, intermittent fever, malaise, and superficial discharge are common features. In chronic discharging lesions there may be transformation of the drainage sinus lining to squamous cell carcinoma (Marjolin's ulcer).

Imaging Features

All the features of acute osteomyelitis can be present. Key features suggesting chronicity are the long length of bony involvement, prominent periosteal involucrum, sclerosis, and sequestra formation. These may best be appreciated on CT scan. The site of discharge from the bone (cloaca) may be identified on CT.

Brodie's Abscess (Bone Abscess, Aborted Osteomyelitis)

Clinical Features

The tibia and femur are the most common sites for this lesion. Pain is the predominant feature; it tends to be chronic and worse at night and may respond to aspirin, mimicking the presentation of osteoid osteoma. Brodie's abscess is a localized infection of bone that is contained by bone response. It may or may not have pus, and frequently no organism is cultured.

Imaging Features

The metaphysis and, less commonly, the epiphysis are the primary sites. In young patients the abscess can be seen to traverse the growth plate. Its shape is variable, from round to oval and occasionally serpiginous. The lesion is geographic in appearance; there is usually a distinct sclerotic border, which can be minimal or extensive (Figure 4–56). In large medullary or small cortical lesions there may be accompanying periosteal new bone. All these features frequently make differentiation from osteoid osteoma and other tumors difficult.

Septic Arthritis (Joint Infection)

Clinical Features

The knee is swollen, hot, and tender. Systemic features of fever and malaise are common. A history of intraarticular infection, surgery, or traumatic intrusion my be evident. Aspiration is necessary for diagnosis.

Imaging Features

Joint effusion is usually the only feature. With progression, loss of the articular plate and diminution of joint space ensue (Figure 4–57). Moth-eaten destruction of the epiphysis may

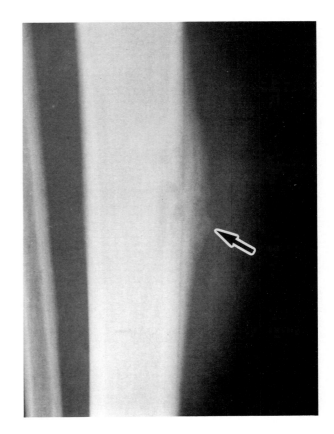

A

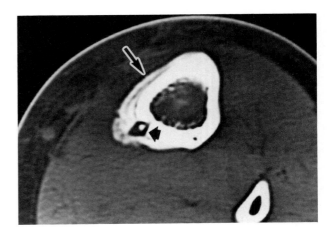

B

Figure 4–55 Acute osteomyelitis. (**A**) Plain film. On the medial cortex of the tibia, note the localized laminated periosteal response (arrow). There is some underlying destruction of the cortex. (**B**) CT scan. On bone window, note the laminated periosteal response (arrow). A small bony sequestrum is also evident (arrowhead). *Comment*: Acute osteomyelitis in its earliest phases is best detected by nuclear bone scan. CT is particularly well suited for defining the extent of the infection.

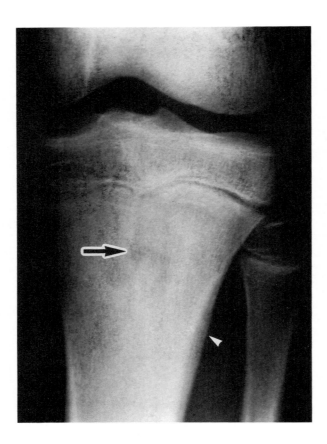

Figure 4–56 Brodie's abscess. Within the proximal tibial metaphysis, a poorly defined geographic defect is visible (arrow). There is also some marginal sclerosis and laminated periosteal new bone at the lateral metaphysis (arrowhead). *Comment*: Brodie's abscess is common in children and adolescents; the tibia is the most common bone affected.

begin to appear coincident with metaphyseal periostitis. Resolution of the infection is often by joint ankylosis.

METABOLIC DISORDERS

Osteoporosis (Osteopenia)

Clinical Features

Loss of bone density is best described as osteopenia unless a cause is known, in which case the correct term is applied. There are many causes of osteopenia, including endocrine imbalance, infections, and neoplastic and posttraumatic abnormalities, among others. The most common causes include postmenopausal hormone changes, immobilization, and trauma.

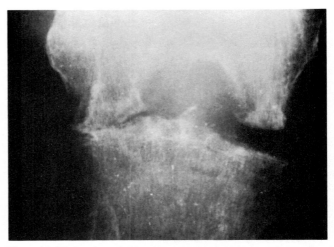

Figure 4–57 Septic arthritis. Observe the destruction of the opposing articular surfaces at both medial and lateral joint compartments. In this case of tuberculous arthritis, there has been widening of the intercondylar notch. *Comment*: Characteristic of joint infections is their ability to destroy both sides of an articulation. Healing is by bony ankylosis if the damage is severe.

Imaging Features

Generally there is diminished bone density, thinning of the cortex, and, depending on severity, accentuation or loss of selected stress-bearing trabeculae. In acute immobilization of a previously healthy bone, there is initially prominent loss of the subarticular bone that spreads rapidly into the epiphysis and metaphysis (Figure 4–58). Osteopenia associated with neoplasm or infection may show moth-eaten, permeative, or geographic destruction and periosteal new bone.

Paget's Disease (Osteitis Deformans)

Paget's disease may affect up to 3% of individuals older than 50 years; the incidence increases to more than 5% by the eighth decade of life. Strong racial and geographic influences exist in that the disease is most common in England and Australia, less common in North America, and rare in Scandinavia and Asia.[54] Much speculation has been made concerning its etiology, but no definitive cause has been delineated.

Clinical Features

The knee is a common site of Paget's disease. The femur is the second most common bone to be involved after the pelvis. The tibia is the fourth most common site, and patellar and fibular locations are considered rare. Notably, in the majority of cases no external signs of underlying Paget's disease will be apparent, and pain is often absent. The disease usually is dis-

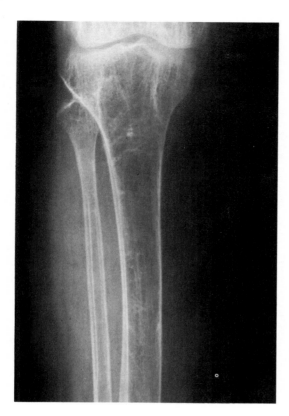

Figure 4–58 Disuse osteoporosis. This patient was virtually immobile for many years. The features of osteopenia are well displayed: thinning of the cortex, decreased bone density, and sparse trabeculae. *Comment*: Such osteopenia can be due to a number of causes, including immobility, corticosteroids, tumor, and endocrine disease.

covered only fortuitously by radiography. External manifestations, however, may include increased overlying skin temperature, visible deformity, vascular bruit, pathologic fracture, and, rarely, a soft tissue mass due to malignant transformation. The major biochemical marker is the alkaline phosphatase enzyme, which fluctuates with disease activity and at times may be remarkably elevated (up to 40 times normal).

Imaging Features

Paget's disease is characterized by the wide diversity of imaging signs. It is a slowly evolving, dynamic disease process that passes through up to four stages: osteolytic, mixed, osteoblastic, and malignant transformation. Consequently, it has been labeled a great imitator of bone disease because of its ability to mimic many other disorders, such as metastatic carcinoma and osteomyelitis. The key signs include cortical thickening, coarse trabeculae, pseudofractures, bone expansion, altered density (lucent, sclerotic, or mixed), and a tendency to begin at one end of the bone and to progress longi-

tudinally to involve the entire bone. Also, early in its evolution the disease conspicuously affects the subarticular bone, which is a key manifestation when this diagnosis is being considered. Isotopic bone scans demonstrate active uptake in all phases of the disease (Figure 4–59).

Femur. It is most common for the disease to begin in the proximal femur and to progress distally. At the normal–pathologic bone interface of the advancing changes, a discrete, radiolucent, V-shaped density may be visible (blade of grass appearance). The diaphyseal-metaphyseal cortex is thickened to involve the articular plate. The trabeculae are coarse and follow trabecular lines. Expansion in bone caliber may be apparent at the femoral condyles. Within the subarticular zone the most common manifestation is an admixture of sclerosis and lucency, which can simulate aggressive destruction or avascular necrosis. Late in the course of the disease lateral bowing of the femur, when combined with coxa vara, can produce a shepherd's crook deformity.

Pseudofractures are most frequent at the lateral and anterior cortices below the trochanters. These are recognizable as linear lucencies with sclerotic margins lying perpendicular to the cortex and associated with a localized bulge at their endosteal surfaces.

Tibia. The disease begins more frequently in the proximal tibia rather than distally. The features are identical to those in the femur. It is, however, more likely to give rise to a blade of grass appearance in the tibia than in any other bone. Early involvement may begin in the tibial tuberosity, producing an ovoid cystic lesion.[54] The major bowing deformity develops anteriorly (sabre shin), which also coincides with the location of pseudofractures.

Fibula. Various reports attest to the rarity of fibular involvement in Paget's disease.[54]

Patella. The patella is an unusual site for Paget's disease. There is often profound enlargement and cortical thickening, and frequently the disease is complicated by transverse fractures.

Complications

A number of secondary problems can occur, some of which can be life threatening.[54]

Sarcomatous Transformation (Paget's Sarcoma). The incidence of secondary malignant tumors is approximately 1%. The most common such tumor is osteosarcoma, although fibrosarcoma and chondrosarcoma do arise on occasion. The femur is a favored site for these tumors, and spread tends to be diaphyseal. Osteosarcoma is readily recognizable by cortical disruption, moth-eaten destruction or a frankly sclerotic reaction, a spiculated periosteal response, and a soft tissue mass

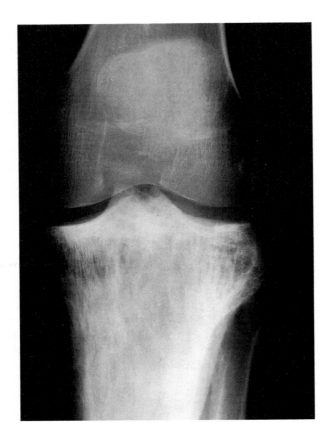

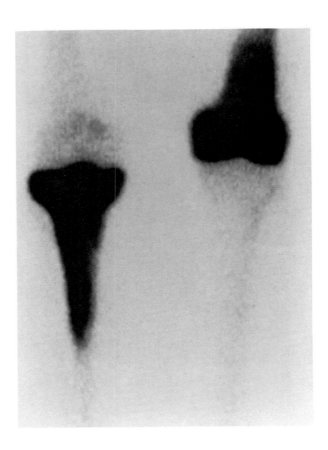

A   B

Figure 4–59 Paget's disease. (**A**) Tibia. There is an increase in bone density of the tibia, accentuation of the trabeculae, cortical thickening, and bone expansion. (**B**) Bone scan. Observe the increased isotope uptake in the femur and contralateral tibia. *Comment:* Paget's disease exhibits these characteristic features and most notably extends to the subarticular bone.

---

that may contain dense sarcomatous bone (cumulus cloud appearance) (Figure 4–60). Clinically these tumors are marked by the appearance of a soft tissue mass, pain, and a rising alkaline phosphatase level. This is usually a lethal complication.

Giant Cell Tumor. GCTs are a rare association. Approximately 25% are frankly malignant. The imaging findings consist of an expansile, epiphyseal-metaphyseal geographic lesion.

Fracture and Deformity. The bone most commonly fractured in Paget's disease is the femur. The femoral locations occur, in descending order of frequency, at the subtrochanteric region (33%), middle third (20%), upper third (15%), femoral

neck (12%), lower third (11%), and the trochanters (9%).[54] These fractures tend to be transverse (banana fracture) and heal within prolific callus, which itself is Pagetic in nature (Figure 4–61). Avulsion of the tibial tuberosity may occur with no associated trauma. Bowing of the femoral and tibial shafts (shepherd's crook and sabre shin deformities) occurs secondary to bone softening and can produce shortening of the limb.

Degenerative Joint Disease. Paget's disease can precipitate degenerative changes by altering the stress biomechanics at the joint as a result of deformity, diminishing support for joint cartilage, and spread of the pathologic process from the subchondral bone to affect the cartilage directly.

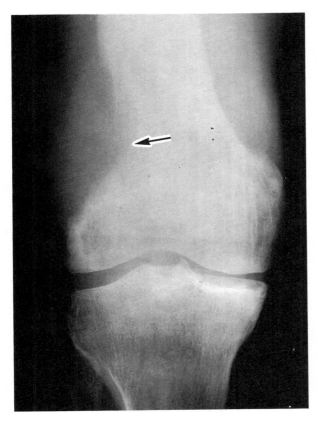

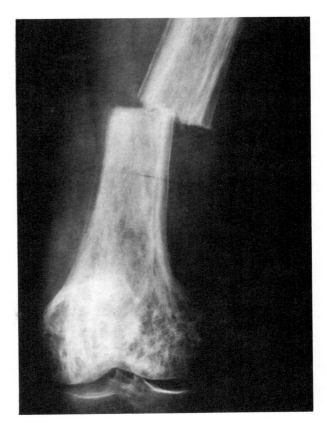

Figure 4–60 Paget's disease, sarcomatous transformation. Observe the characteristic Paget's disease of the distal femur. There is, however, destruction of the lateral cortex (arrow) with an associated soft tissue mass. *Comment:* Paget's sarcoma is a rare complication but tends to involve the femur.

Figure 4–61 Paget's disease, banana fracture. Discrete bone changes of Paget's disease are clearly seen in the distal femur. Observe the transverse pathologic fracture in the distal femoral shaft. *Comment:* Bone softening in Paget's disease predisposes to these fractures.

REFERENCES

1. Leach RE, Gregg T, Ferris JS. Weight-bearing radiography in osteoarthritis of the knee. *Radiology.* 1970; 97:265.

2. Thomas RH, Resnick D, Alazraki NP, Daniel D, Greenfield R. Compartmental evaluation of osteoarthritis of the knee. A comparative study of available diagnostic modalities. *Radiology.* 1975; 116:585.

3. Weissman BNW, Sledge CB. The knee. In: Weissman BNW, Sledge CB, eds. *Orthopedic Radiology.* Philadelphia: Saunders; 1986:497.

4. Rosenburg TD, Paulos LE, Parker RD, Coward DB, Scott SM. The forty-five-degree posteroanterior flexion weight-bearing radiograph of the knee. *J Bone Joint Surg Am.* 1988; 70:1479.

5. Homblad EC. Postero-anterior X-ray view of the knee in flexion. *JAMA.* 1937; 109:1196.

6. Rowe LJ, Yochum TR. Hematologic and vascular disease of bone. In: Yochum TR, Rowe LJ, eds. *Essentials of Skeletal Radiology.* Baltimore: Williams & Wilkins; 1987.

7. Wiberg G. Roentgenographic and anatomic studies on the patellofemoral joint. *Acta Orthop Scand.* 1941; 12:916.

8. Hughston JC. Subluxation of the patella. *J Bone Joint Surg Am.* 1968; 50: 1003.

9. Knutsson F. Uber die rentgenologie des hemoropatellargelenks sowie enine gute projektion fur das kniegelenk. *Acta Radiol.* 1941; 22:371.

10. Merchant AC, Mercer RL, Jacobsen RH, Cool CR. Roentgenologic analysis of the patellofemoral joint congruence. *J Bone Joint Surg Am.* 1974; 56:1391.

11. Laurin CA, Dussault R, Levesque HP. The tangential X-ray investigation of the patellofemoral joint: X-ray technique, diagnostic criteria and their interpretation. *Clin Orthop Rel Res.* 1979; 144:16.

12. Langer JE, Meyer SJF, Dalinka MK. Imaging of the knee. *Radiol Clin North Am.* 1990; 28:975.

13. Kursunoglu S, Pate D, Resnick D, et al. Computer arthrotomography with multiplanar reformations and three-dimensional image analysis in the evaluation of the cruciate ligaments: preliminary investigation. *J Can Assoc Radiol.* 1986; 37:153.

14. Genant H. Computed tomography. In: Resnick D, Niwayama G, eds. *Diagnosis of Bone and Joint Disorders*. Philadelphia: Saunders; 1981:380.

15. Mink JH, Deutsch AL. The knee. In: Mink JH, Deutsch AL, eds. *MRI of the Musculoskeletal System. A Teaching File*. New York: Raven; 1990:330.

16. Alazraki N. Bone imaging by radionuclide techniques. In: Resnick D, Niwayama G, eds. *Diagnosis of Bone and Joint Disorders*. Philadelphia: Saunders; 1981:639.

17. Insall J, Salvata E. Patella position in the normal knee joint. *Radiology*. 1971; 101:101.

18. Vainionpaa S, Laike E, Kirves P, Tiusanen P. Tibial osteotomy for osteoarthritis of the knee. *J Bone Joint Surg Am*. 1981; 63:938.

19. Keats TE, Lusted LB. *An Atlas of Roentgenographic Measurements*. 5th ed. Chicago: Year Book Medical; 1985.

20. Lindahl O, Movin A. Roentgenologic angulation measurement in supracondylar fractures of the femur. *Acta Radiol (Diagn)*. 1970; 10:108.

21. Jacobsen K. Radiologic technique for measuring instability in the knee joint. *Acta Radiol (Diagn)*. 1974; 18:113.

22. Blank N, Liever A. The significance of growing bone islands. *Radiology*. 1965; 85:508.

23. Onitsuka H. Roentgenologic aspects of bone islands. *Radiology*. 1977; 123:607.

24. Davies JA, Hall FM, Goldberg RP, et al. Positive bone scans in bone islands. *J Bone Joint Surg Am*. 1979; 61:6.

25. Kohler A, Zimmer EA. *Borderlands of the Normal and Early Pathologic in Skeletal Roentgenology*. San Diego: Grune & Stratton; 1968.

26. Weaver JK. Bipartite patella as a cause of disability in the athlete. *Am J Sports Med*. 1977; 5:137.

27. Lawson JP. Not-so-normal variants. *Orthop Clin North Am*. 1990; 21:483.

28. George R. Bilateral bipartite patella. *Br J Surg*. 1935; 22:555.

29. Ogden JA, McCarthy SM, Jokl P. The painful bipartite patella. *J Pediatr Orthop*. 1982; 2:263.

30. Echeverria TS, Bersini FA. Acute fracture simulating a symptomatic bipartite patella. *Am J Sports Med*. 1980; 8:48.

31. van Holsbeek M, Vandamme B, Marchal G, et al. Dorsal defect of the patella. Concept of its origin and relationship with bipartite and multipartite patella. *Skeletal Radiol*. 1987; 16:304.

32. Johnson JF, Brogden BG. Dorsal defect of the patella; incidence and distribution. *AJR*. 1982; 139:339.

33. Denham RH. Dorsal defect of the patella. *J Bone Joint Surg Am*. 1984; 66:116.

34. Haswell DM, Berne AS, Graham CB. The dorsal defect of the patella. *Pediatr Radiol*. 1976; 4:238.

35. Georgen TG, Resnick D, Greenway G. Dorsal defect of the patella (DDP): a characteristic radiographic lesion. *Radiology*. 1979; 130:333.

36. Ho VB, Kransdorf MJ, Jelinek JS, et al. Dorsal defect of the patella: MR features. *J Comput Assisted Tomogr*. 1991; 15:474.

37. Harrison RB. The grooves of the distal articular surface of the femur—a normal variant. *AJR*. 1976; 126:751.

38. Caffey J. Ossification of the distal femoral epiphysis. *J Bone Joint Surg Am*. 1958; 41:647.

39. Burrows PE. The distal femoral defect: technetium-99m pyrophosphate bone scan results. *J Can Assoc Radiol*. 1982; 33:91.

40. Keats TE. The distal anterior metaphyseal defect: an anatomic variant that may simulate disease. *AJR* 1974; 121:101.

41. Levine AH. The soleal line: a cause of tibial pseudoperiostitis. *Radiology*. 1976; 119:79.

42. Pitt MJ. Radiology of the femoral linea aspera–pilaster complex: the track sign. *Radiology*. 1982; 142:66.

43. Weber WN, Neumann CH, Barakos JA, et al. Lateral tibial rim (Segond) fractures: MR imaging characteristics. *Radiology*. 1991; 180:731.

44. Rowe LJ. Metatarsal stress fracture. *ACA Counc Roentgenol Briefs*. 1982.

45. Daffner RH. Stress fractures: current concepts. *Skeletal Radiol*. 1978; 2:221.

46. Symeonides PP. High stress fracture of the fibula. *J Bone Joint Surg Br*. 1980; 62:192.

47. Kransdorf MJ, Meis JM, Jelinek JS. Myositis ossificans: MR appearance with radiologic–pathologic correlation. *AJR*. 1991; 157:1243.

48. Li DKB, Adams ME, McConkey JP. Magnetic resonance imaging of the ligaments and menisci of the knee. *Radiol Clin North Am*. 1986; 24:209.

49. Fairbanks TJ. Knee joint changes after meniscectomy. *J Bone Joint Surg Br*. 1948; 30:664.

50. Ogden JA, Southwick WO. Osgood-Schlatter disease and tibial tuberosity development. *Clin Orthop Rel Res*. 1976; 116:180.

51. De Smet AA, Fisher DR, Graf BK, Lange RH. Osteochondritis dissecans of the knee: value of MR imaging in determining lesion stability and the presence of articular cartilage defects. *AJR*. 1990; 155:549.

52. Greenspan A, Norman, A, Tchang FK. "Tooth" sign in patella degenerative disease. *J Bone Joint Surg Am*. 1977; 59:483.

53. McCauley TR, Kier R, Lynch KJ, Jokl P. Chondromalacia patellae: diagnosis with MR imaging. *AJR*. 1992; 158:101.

54. Wilner D. *Radiology of Bone Tumors and Allied Disorders*. Philadelphia: Saunders; 1982.

55. Enzinger FM, Harvey DA. Spindle cell lipoma. *Cancer*. 1975; 36:1852.

56. Tilman BP, Dahlin DC, Lipscomb PR, et al. Aneurysmal bone cyst: an analysis of ninety five cases. *Mayo Clin Proc*. 1968; 43:478.

57. Chan O, Thomas ML. The incidence of popliteal aneurysms in patients with ateriomegaly. *Clin Radiol*. 1990; 41:185.

58. Lotke PA, Abend JA, Ecker ML. The treatment of osteonecrosis of the medial femoral condyle. *Clin Orthop*. 1982; 171:109.

59. Bonakdarpour A, Millmond SLT, Mesgarzadeh M. Spontaneous osteonecrosis of the knee. *Contemp Diagn Radiol*. 1987; 10:1.

60. Munk PL, Helms CA, Holt RG. Immature bone infarcts: findings on plain radiographs and MR scans. *AJR*. 1989; 152:547.

61. Schauwecker DS. The scintographic diagnosis of osteomyelitis. *AJR*. 1992; 158:9.

62. Murray RO, Jacobsen HG. *The Radiology of Skeletal Disorders*. 2nd ed. New York: Churchill Livingstone; 1977.

Chapter 5

Adjustive Techniques

Egyptologists have suggested that the ancient Egyptians were performing manipulations before the time of Christ. Other cultures that used manipulation in one form or another include the Greek physicians, native Americans, eastern Europeans, and the Japanese.

Andrew Still linked manipulation to the principles of osteopathy and started the first osteopathic school in 1874 at Kirksville, Missouri. DD Palmer in 1895 founded the principles of chiropractic. He did not claim the discovery of manipulation, but he did claim to be the first to use the spinous and transverse processes of the vertebrae as levers to adjust specific vertebrae. Palmer founded the first chiropractic college in 1897 at Davenport, Iowa.

Palmer referred to adjusting the 300 articulations of the body, which included the extremities as well as the spine and pelvis. Over the years the philosophy of some schools and some political entities have placed restrictions on the areas to be manipulated, but the profession as a whole encompasses manipulation of all the articulations as accepted practice. When dysfunction exists in an extremity that may be related to a fixation of the spine or pelvis, all fixations of the spine and pelvis should be corrected before the extremity problem is addressed, where possible.

Most of the adjustive techniques in this book are based on those developed by Metzinger[1] and taught to the author by Crawford and Metzinger. Alternative techniques are shown where appropriate. Within our profession as well as osteopathy, many techniques have been developed and used successfully. I have reviewed *Athletic and Industrial Injuries of the Knee*[2] by Schultz, some of whose techniques I have used and/or adapted, and *Atlas of Osteopathic Techniques*[3] by Nicholas.

With the announcement that I was in the process of writing a book about the knee, numerous sets of notes on technique were provided from around the world for my review. I have also attended many seminars on techniques involving the knee by many different proponents. The techniques that follow are what I have found the most useful in practice.

LATERALLY ROTATED TIBIA ON THE FEMUR

Signs and Symptoms

The patient may be asymptomatic or may exhibit a variety of symptoms from knee ache to the inability to walk. The patient may be unable to extend the knee fully. The condition may be associated with a tight iliotibial tract and biceps.

Tests

The medial condyle of the tibia fails to move anteriorly from under the femur during hyperextension. Palpate the anterior surface of the medial condyle of both the femur and the tibia (Figure 5–1). Elevate the ankle to produce hyperextension. Failure of the medial tibial condyle to move anteriorly from under the femoral condyle indicates a fixation.

Another test for laterally rotated tibia fixation is as follows. With the femur secured, apply pressure posteriorly on the me-

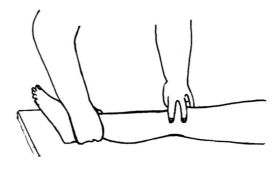

A

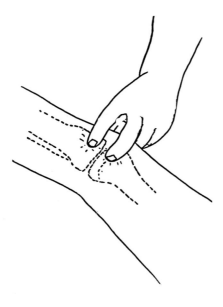

B

Figure 5–1 (**A** and **B**) Right knee, contacts for palpation of medial condyle motion.

dial tibial condyle (Figure 5–2). If the fixation exists, no movement will be felt.

During the examination, there are two signs of a possible tibial rotation. Upon flexing the knee, the heel may align itself medial to the ischial tuberosity (Figure 5–3), or lateral mobility may be restricted (Figure 5–4).

Precautions and Contraindications

If the patient is unable to flex completely, an alternative technique should be used. The technique should not be used with any degree of instability or if hemarthrosis is present. Execution of the technique should never allow movement beyond the normal range of motion.

Adjustive Technique

While palpating the anterior knee joint with the supporting hand, grasp the ankle and flex the knee, moving the heel near

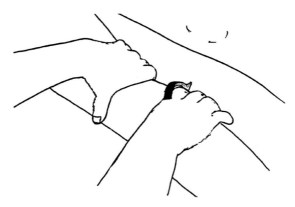

Figure 5–2 Right knee, palpation and adjustment for lateral rotation fixation.

the buttocks (Figure 5–5). Rotate the tibia medially while abducting (Figure 5–6). After abduction and rotation, return the ankle to approximately 30° of flexion (Figure 5–7). All the above should be executed quickly and smoothly as one movement, keeping within the normal range of motion. A clicking may be heard and should be felt by the supporting hand if correction is made. Extension should not exceed 30°. There should not be any whipping of the leg at the end.

Caution should always be used in a trauma case where edema and/or hemarthrosis is present because the fluid pres-

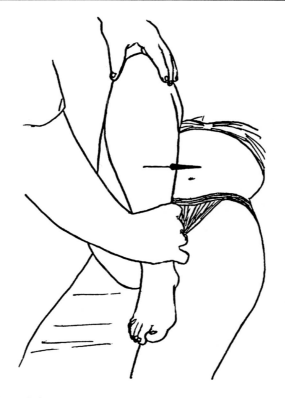

Figure 5–3 Right knee, flexion with medial heel alignment.

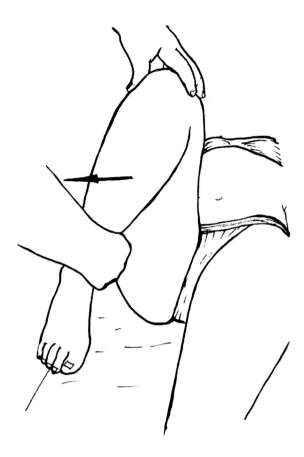

Figure 5–4 Right knee, restricted lateral mobility.

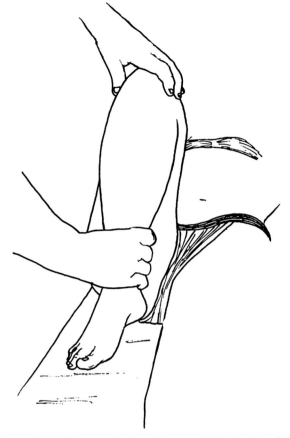

Figure 5–5 Adjustment for laterally rotated tibia fixation, first part.

sure may cloud an instability in normal testing procedures. Staying within the normal range of motion is necessary to protect the knee.

The laterally rotated tibia is the most common fixation of the knee. If present, it should be corrected and then the other fixations repalpated.

With any fixation, the muscles involved that would either produce it or allow it to occur must be considered. The biceps and the iliotibial tract are the only lateral rotators, and then only with the knee flexed. Medial rotation is produced by the popliteus muscle in all ranges of extension and flexion and is assisted by the medial hamstrings, sartorius, and gracilis in the flexed knee.

Several authors of medical texts suggest a manipulation similar to this adjustment. They refer to the popping or click as torn, dislocated, or "heaped up" meniscus slipping back into place and consider this a useful way of unlocking the knee.[4,5] A dislocated or "heaped up" meniscus would not be present if the bone structure were properly aligned. Correction of a laterally rotated tibia is a vital step in allowing the soft tissues of the knee joint to repair rapidly and return to normal function, whether the meniscus is torn, "heaped up," or just stretched.

After adjusting the laterally rotated tibia, any muscles that tested weak should be retested. The fixation may interfere with normal function of any of the muscles that cross the joint.

The examination to determine the possibility of an anatomic short leg may be clouded in the presence of this fixation. Lateral rotation alters bone position that either is caused by muscle imbalance or may produce a muscle reaction. All the above interfere with palpation of the end of the femur as a landmark and may disturb the overall distance from the hip to the medial malleolus.

Alternative Technique 1

If complete flexion is not possible, place the patient's ankle on your shoulder nearest the table. With the inside hand (primary contact), grasp the anterior surface of the medial tibial condyle with a pisiform hook contact. Lace the fingers together with the outside hand supporting the knee (Figure 5–8). The thrust is a pull on the pisiform contact toward the floor with medial rotation.

Caution: If edema and/or hemarthrosis is present, care must be taken to ensure that no further damage occurs. The thrust

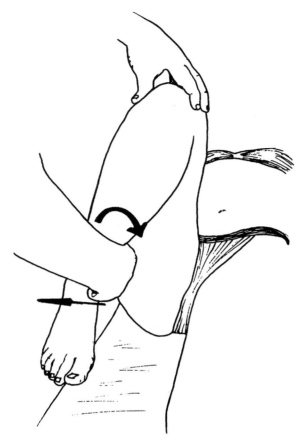

Figure 5–6 Adjustment for laterally rotated tibia fixation, second part.

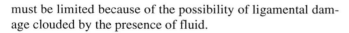

Figure 5–7 Adjustment for laterally rotated tibia fixation, third part.

must be limited because of the possibility of ligamental damage clouded by the presence of fluid.

Alternative Technique 2

With the headward hand, grasp the medial condyle of the femur, and laterally rotate the knee while slightly flexing the knee. Using an index contact on the anterior surface of the medial tibial condyle, thrust posteriorly with some rotation (Figure 5–9).

Alternative Technique 3

This is a technique for minimal fixations that may only exist as a result of a stretched muscle. It may also be useful for the patient in whom adjusting might be either painful or contraindicated.

Place the patient supine with the hip and knee flexed. Secure the foot, preventing its movement into medial rotation. Have the patient attempt medial rotation (Figure 5–10). Gently at first (and if little or no pain is present) increase the strength of the attempt, and release. Repeat several times until the pain diminishes and the attempt becomes stronger. The

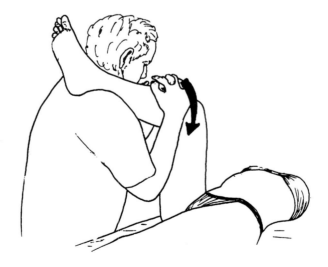

Figure 5–8 Alternative adjustment for laterally rotated tibia fixation.

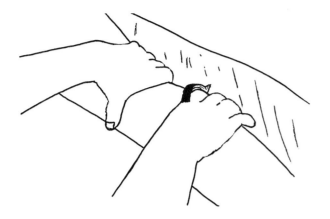

Figure 5–9 Right knee, palpation and adjustment for lateral rotation fixation.

exercise is simply to restore muscle function and to establish patient confidence that the muscle may perform.

If pain is present and fails to reduce or disappear after three exertions, stop the exercise and reevaluate.

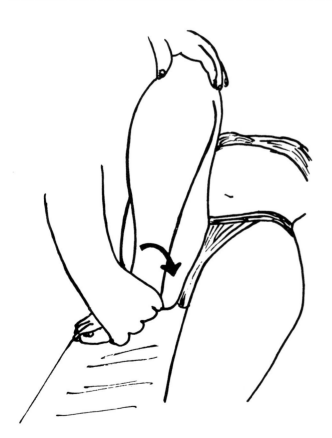

Figure 5–10 Alternative technique for minimal fixation.

MEDIALLY ROTATED TIBIA ON THE FEMUR

This fixation seldom occurs. The muscles that produce lateral rotation (biceps and iliotibial tract) would have to be strained or the medial hamstrings and popliteus would have to be in contraction to produce the fixation. If the fixation should occur, the adjustive technique is the opposite of the laterally rotated fixation technique.

ANTERIOR TIBIA FIXATION ON THE FEMUR

The anterior fixation is usually associated with a laterally rotated tibia fixation. If it is corrected, the anterior fixation is usually corrected along with it. If not, place a rolled towel under the femoral condyles. Reinforce a web contact on the tibial condyles, being careful to avoid a femoral head contact, and thrust posteriorly (Figure 5–11).

By altering the technique slightly using an index contact on the medial tibial condyle, this technique may be used as another alternative technique for the laterally rotated tibia fixation.

POSTERIOR TIBIA FIXATION ON THE FEMUR

Place a rolled towel under the tibial condyles. Use a reinforced web contact on the femur condyles, thrusting posteriorly (Figure 5–12).

Alternatively, with the patient prone use a bilateral pisiform hook contact on the tibial condyles. The thrust is a sharp pull toward the end of the table (Figure 5–13).

LATERAL TIBIA FIXATION ON THE FEMUR

Usually this is found with lateral rotation fixations. If so, correct the lateral rotation first and then palpate again. A combination of weakened vastus medialis oblique fibers, popliteus, and medial hamstrings and a shortened or con-

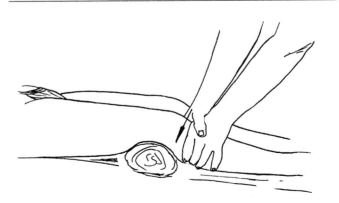

Figure 5–11 Adjustment for anterior tibia fixation.

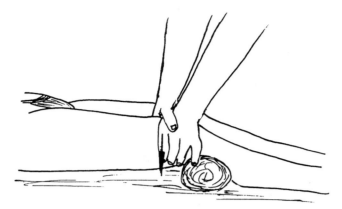

Figure 5–12 Adjustment for posterior tibia fixation.

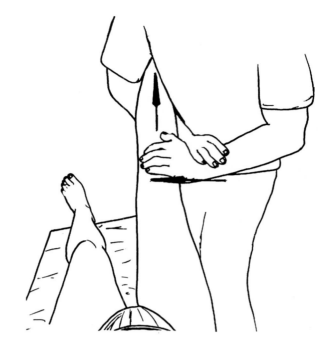

Figure 5–14 Adjustment for lateral tibia fixation.

tracted biceps, iliotibial tract, and vastus lateralis may contribute to producing a lateral tibia fixation.

Secure the patient's ankle under the operator's arm. Use a pisiform contact of the outside hand on the lateral tibial condyle (be careful to avoid the fibula head). Secure the contact hand by placing the inside arm under the leg and the hand over the wrist. This allows complete control of the knee (Figure 5–14).

Flex the knee slightly and, using moderate traction, thrust medially. *This is a limited thrust* and should never be necessary, nor should it be used, if medial instability is found or suspected during the examination.

As an alternative technique, place the foot between operator's knees and traction the leg. Use an index contact on the lateral tibial condyle while supporting the medial femoral condyle with the opposite hand. Slightly flex the knee and, using moderate traction, thrust medially on the tibial condyle with the opposite hand offering resistance to the femur (Figure

5–15). Again, this is a *limited thrust* and should never be necessary, nor should it be used, if medial instability is found or suspected.

MEDIAL TIBIA FIXATION ON THE FEMUR

This is not a common fixation, and when found it is usually associated with a rotated tibia, which if corrected usually removes both fixations.

Secure the patient's ankle under the operator's arm. Use a pisiform contact of the inside hand on the medial tibial

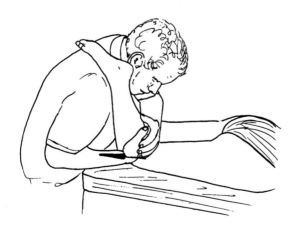

Figure 5–13 Adjustment for posterior tibia fixation, patient in prone position.

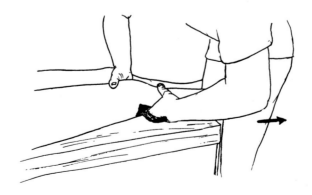

Figure 5–15 Adjustment for lateral tibia fixation, alternative technique.

condyle. Secure the contact hand by placing the outside arm under the leg and the hand over the wrist. This allows complete control of the knee (Figure 5–16). Flex the knee slightly and, using moderate traction, thrust laterally. *This is a limited thrust* and should never be necessary, nor should it be used, if lateral instability is found or suspected during the examination.

Alternatively, place the patient's foot between operator's knees and traction the leg. Use an index contact on the medial tibial condyle while supporting the lateral femoral condyle with the opposite hand (Figure 5–17). Slightly flex the knee and, using moderate traction, thrust laterally on the tibial condyle with the opposite hand offering resistance to the femur. Again, this is a *limited thrust* and should never be necessary, nor should it be used, if lateral instability is found or suspected.

POSTERIOR FIBULA HEAD FIXATION

Place the patient in the prone position with the knee flexed to 90° and the ankle resting against the operator's shoulder (see Figure 5–18). Use a pisiform hook contact of the outside hand around the fibula head reinforced with the support hand. Rotate the fibula head anterolaterally and thrust with a sharp, shallow pull (take care not to pinch the lateral head of the gastrocnemius muscle).

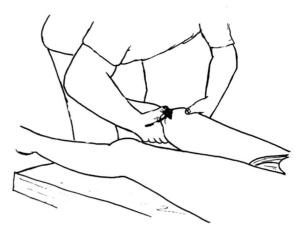

Figure 5–17 Adjustment for medial tibia fixation, alternative technique.

Alternative Technique 1

With the patient in the prone position and the leg extended, slightly rotate the leg laterally. Stabilize the leg with the support hand (Figure 5–19). Using a pisiform contact on the posterior aspect of the fibula head, give a quick, shallow thrust following the articular plane anterolaterally.

Alternative Technique 2

With the patient supine, place the ankle between the operator's knees and apply mild traction (only to stabilize). With the inside hand, grasp medial and anterior knee structures to prevent anterior movement. With the outside hand, use an index finger hook behind the fibula head with the rest of the fingers around the fibula (Figure 5–20). The thrust is a sharp pull anterolaterally.

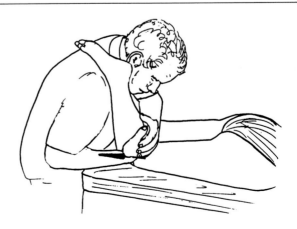

Figure 5–18 Adjustment for posterior tibia fixation, patient in prone position.

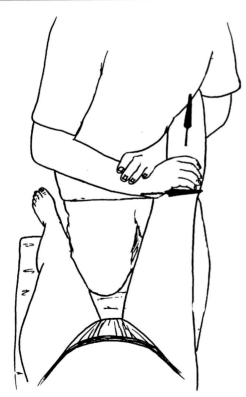

Figure 5–16 Adjustment for medial tibia fixation.

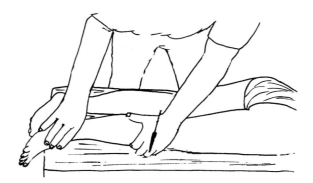

Figure 5–19 Adjustment for posterior fibula head fixation.

SUPERIOR FIBULA HEAD FIXATION

A superior fibula head fixation occurs from a hypertonic biceps femoris muscle and/or weakness of the fibula and foot muscles (peroneus longus, brevis, and tertius; flexor hallucis longus; extensor hallucis longus; extensor digitorum longus; soleus; and posterior tibialis).

With the patient in the prone position, medially rotate the leg by rotating the heel out with the support hand. From the opposite side of the table, contact the fibula head with a pisiform contact on the headward hand (Figure 5–21). The thrust is shallow and as inferior as possible.

ANTERIOR FIBULA HEAD FIXATION

With the patient in the supine position, support the ankle with the footward hand. Using a pisiform contact on the anterior fibula head, thrust posteroinferiorly on the fibula head (Figure 5–22).

INFERIOR FIBULA HEAD FIXATION

With the patient in the prone position and the knee flexed, dorsiflex the ankle by bracing it against the chest. While ap-

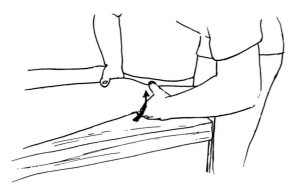

Figure 5–20 Adjustment for posterior fibula head fixation, alternative technique.

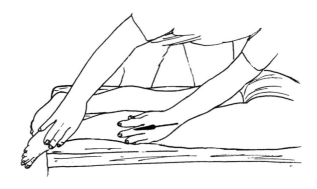

Figure 5–21 Adjustment for superior fibula head fixation.

plying dorsiflexion, contact the fibula head with both thumbs. The thrust is made by using the operator's body weight to dorsiflex the ankle farther while thrusting with both thumbs toward the table (Figure 5–23).

SUPERIOR PATELLA FIXATION

Although not a fixation of an articulation, this is a common finding that may be corrected readily in most cases.

With the leg extended, simply hold the patella firmly with a web contact, push inferiorly, and hold until the quadriceps relaxes (Figure 5–24).

This is especially effective in older patients who have stopped flexing the knee (by squatting and similar movements), in whom the quadriceps becomes either shortened or hypertonic. Older patients who have had knee pain and have received cortisone injections often end up with contracted quadriceps muscles that interfere with normal function of the knee.

Caution: The presence of chondromalacia in the elderly is common (it may be the reason for the use of cortisone). Not

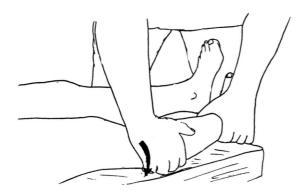

Figure 5–22 Adjustment for anterior fibula head fixation.

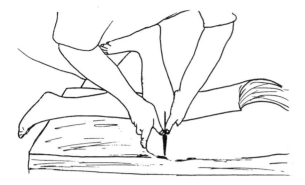

Figure 5–23 Adjustment for inferior fibula head fixation.

only should the diagnosis be made first, but caution should be used not to apply posterior pressure during the stretch. Follow-up therapy should include stretching exercises at home.

MEDIAL MENISCUS ENTRAPMENT

After all other adjustments are made, repalpate. If palpation reveals a small nodule or nodules along the medial joint line, an entrapment should be considered. Usually the nodule is extremely tender as a result of a small tear of the medial capsular ligament allowing the entrapment of a small portion of the meniscus.

With valgus trauma to the knee, the medial joint space may be stressed beyond the normal limits, causing the tear. Upon returning to its normal position, the joint space entraps the meniscus, leaving a small protrusion that feels like a match head under the skin.

With the patient in the supine position, sit on a stool approximately the same height as the table facing footward.

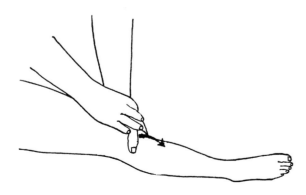

Figure 5–24 Adjustment for superior patella fixation (quadriceps femoris stretch).

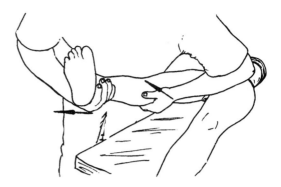

Figure 5–25 Adjustment for medial meniscus entrapment.

With the outside hand, grasp the ankle from underneath. Place the knee firmly against the operator's ilium (this prevents any pressure on the joint). With the fingers around and behind the knee, contact the nodule with a pisiform contact (Figure 5–25).

The protrusion may be anterior or posterior of the midline of the meniscus. The thrust should be made toward the center of the knee joint. Rotate the leg until the thrust is toward both the center of the joint and the operator's ilium.

Traction the ankle laterally, but only as far as necessary to open the medial joint. This may be determined during palpation in preparation for the contact.

The thrust is made toward the center of the knee by the operator placing the elbow at 90° to the ilium. With a correct contact against the ilium, the thrust itself can do no harm to the knee structure. The thrust may be made sharply as the joint opens up by traction on the ankle laterally.

As a follow-up, the author has found 3 minutes of ultrasound at approximately half power effective in promoting healing when coupled with 2 to 3 days of restricted flexion of the knee past 20°.

Although not as effective as the above technique, the following alternative is useful in mild cases. With the patient supine, flex the hip and knee. Rotate the tibia (using the foot) medially. This exposes the medial meniscus for easy palpation (Figure 5–26A). Apply pressure toward the center of the knee with a thumb contact while rotating the tibia laterally and extending the knee (Figure 5–26B).

LATERAL MENISCUS ENTRAPMENT

As in meniscus tears, more meniscus entrapments are found medially than laterally because of the lateral meniscus' mobility and lack of lateral attachments. If suspected (the author has found only one case), the technique is the reverse of the technique described above.

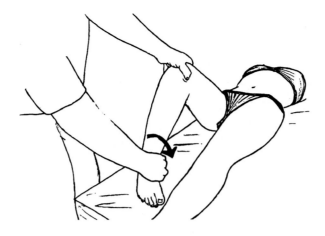

A

Figure 5–26 (A) Contacts for medial meniscus entrapment, alternative technique.

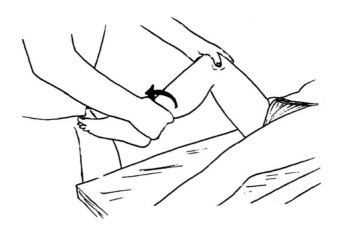

B

Figure 5–26 (B) Adjustment maneuver.

REFERENCES

1. Metzinger DJ. *Technique Notes*. Los Angeles: Hollywood Chiropractic College; 1956.
2. Schultz A. *Athletic and Industrial Injuries of the Knee*. Stickney, SD: Argus; 1963.
3. Nicholas NS. *Atlas of Osteopathic Techniques*. Philadelphia: Philadelphia College of Osteopathic Medicine; 1980.
4. Hoppenfeld S. *Physical Examination of the Spine and Extremities*. New York: Appleton-Century-Crofts; 1976.
5. Kuland DN. *The Injured Athlete*. Philadelphia: Lippincott; 1988.

Chapter 6

Conditions and Therapy

Many texts on the knee deal primarily with severe damage, diagnosis, and the surgical procedures necessary for repair. This chapter addresses problems of the knee all the way from mild postural strain to instability that may be treated conservatively in the office or referred for possible surgery.

CHRONIC KNEE DYSFUNCTION DUE TO POSTURAL STRAIN

Many deviations from normal posture may produce strain to the knee. In the average practice, a majority of patients with knee symptoms have postural faults that either contribute to the problem or are the direct cause of the problem. Any preexisting postural strain becomes a major factor in the recovery from trauma. If not detected, rehabilitation from trauma will be difficult, if not impossible; therefore, the most common postural fault will be covered first.

Lordotic Lumbar Syndrome

Probably the most common source of knee strain is postural stress. Lordotic lumbar syndrome (Figure 6–1) is prevalent in any society where there are conveniences of modern life and the workforce is employed in sitting jobs. Although common in both sexes, it is more prevalent in the female because of the following:

- distortions of the late stage of pregnancy
- wearing of high-heeled shoes

- higher frequency of abdominal surgeries
- wearing of bras, which restricts rib cage elevation during inspiration and the release of the rectus abdominus muscle, allowing the anterior pelvis to drop inferiorly

Stretched or weakened abdominal muscles, whether from pregnancy, surgery, obesity, or just lack of exercise, and regardless of sex, result in anterior rotation of the pelvis, increased lumbar lordosis, increased lumbosacral angle, stretched (and sometimes weakened) gluteus maximus muscles, hypertonic or shortened psoas and iliacus muscles, and stretched and/or weakened piriformis muscles (with weakening of the more powerful gluteus maximus muscles, the piriformis muscles eventually are stretched also).

Medially Rotated Femur and Knee Problems

With weakened or stretched piriformis and gluteal muscles, the femur rotates medially (the trochanters rotate anteriorly; Figure 6–2). In the standing radiograph with the knees not touching and the feet facing forward, medial rotation may be detected by the diminished size of the lesser trochanters and usually an associated valgus knee.

With medial rotation of the femur (Figure 6–3) the normal Q angle (valgus angle) is increased, allowing the following to occur:

- Reduction in the pectineus muscle length and reduction of the femur-pubic space may affect circulation to and from the lower extremity. Often the patient complains of

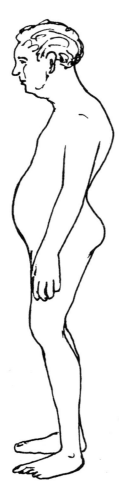

Figure 6–1 Lordotic lumbar syndrome.

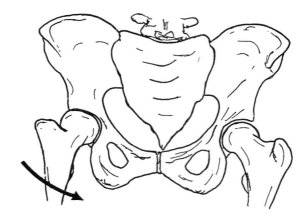

Figure 6–2 Medially rotated femur.

groin pain. Palpation over the pectineus muscle will reproduce the pain (this may also occur in iliopectineus bursitis). To differentiate, manually rotate the pelvis posteriorly. If only a reactive pectineus muscle is present, the pain will disappear. If iliopectineal bursitis exists, the pain will not diminish and may increase.

- The ability of the sartorius muscle to function is reduced.
- The ability of the rectus femoris muscle to function is reduced.
- The valgus angle of the knee is increased.
- Stress is increased on the vastus medialis muscle, especially the oblique fibers (VMO).
- The abnormal tracking of the patella in the trochlear groove may produce inflammation and lead to degeneration.
- The increased Q angle usually produces a compensatory lateral rotation of the tibia.
- The lateral rotation may produce a pronated foot.

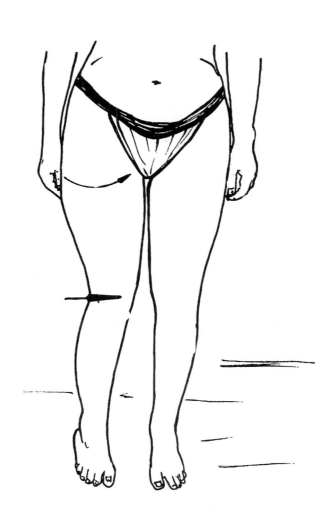

Figure 6–3 Valgus knee and medially rotated femur (increased Q angle).

A common finding in practice is the postpartum woman who after one or more births is unable or unwilling to do the proper exercises to restore abdominal tone. With dysfunction continuing for months and years, she presents with bilateral valgus knees. The valgus knee is not the cause of the problem but a result of the low back and pelvis distortion. Treatment should be addressed to alleviate immediate pain, but the lordotic lumbar syndrome must be the primary target of treatment.

Patients may function for many years with all the stress listed above but with only minimal discomfort or fatigue. Without trauma, major symptoms may not appear until degeneration makes normal movement impossible without pain.

Treatment of the patient with knee symptoms who also has a lordotic lumbar syndrome should include adjustment of all fixations of the foot and ankle, adjustment of all fixations of the spine and pelvis that may relate to the knee and/or the lordotic syndrome, and various exercises as described below.

Exercises for Abdominal Muscles

While lying on the floor with the legs on a chair, the patient attempts sit-ups in 6 positions from the extreme right to the extreme left (Figure 6–4). Each movement should be to reach as far as possible, hold for a moment, and then slowly return to the floor. Sit-up exercises performed rapidly and with bouncing from the floor each time are not as effective.

With the hip flexed to 90° the psoas action is decreased, and most of the action is performed with the abdominal muscles. Usually a portion of the psoas muscle is short or hypertonic in the lordotic lumbar syndrome patient.

The psoas muscle may be stretched using the Thomas test position, flexing the opposite leg with the knee to the chest. The author finds this maneuver usually a waste of time except in the acute case with the psoas muscle in spasm.

Lordosis Exercise

With the patient in the supine position, place 10 to 20 lb of weight on the abdomen below the umbilicus. Flex one knee (Figure 6–5) and with that leg elevate the buttocks from the table while posteriorly rotating the pelvis. Hold for a moment, and then slowly return to the table. Repeat 6 to 8 times. Repeat on the opposite side. Compare one side with the other, and for the side that takes more effort repeat 6 to 8 times.

Exercises for the Gluteus Maximus Muscle

With the patient on all fours and the knee bent, push the foot toward the ceiling (Figure 6–6). Do not extend the hip joint beyond 10°. All movement past 10° must be made with the pelvis and would increase the lordosis.

Exercises for the Piriformis Muscle

In the seated position with the hip at 90° of flexion, the piriformis becomes an abductor of the thigh. Have the patient

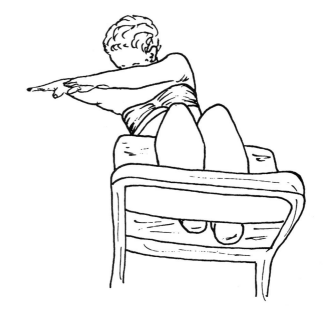

A

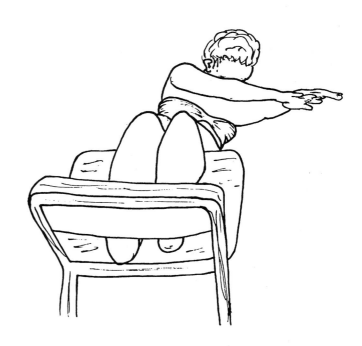

B

Figure 6–4 (A) Far right position for sit-up exercise. **(B)** Far left position for sit-up exercise.

recline back sufficiently to bring hip flexion to approximately 45°. With exercise tubing secured laterally, move the foot medially against resistance, laterally rotating the femur (Figure 6–7).

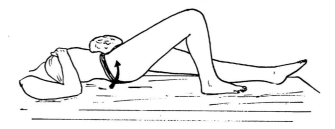

Figure 6–5 Lordosis exercise.

Anatomic Short Leg and Knee Problems

Patients with an anatomic short leg of ¹/₄ in or more will usually have lordotic lumbar syndrome. *It will never respond to exercises* because it is necessary as a part of the compensation for the imbalance. Of course, the case becomes more complicated if compensation exists *and* muscle weakness exists.

The anatomic short leg is further complicated by either of the following[1]:

1. On the short leg side, the patient may laterally rotate the femur, producing a laterally rotated femur fixation and thus a longer leg (another compensation).
2. On the long leg side, the patient may laterally rotate the femur but will widen the stance, attempting to balance the pelvis.

In either case, lateral rotation of the leg produces abnormal function of the foot. The patient may walk Charlie Chaplin-style on the rotated side. This in turn may produce pronation of the foot, further lateral rotation of the tibia, and valgus stress on the knee.

Treatment should include a careful analysis of the anatomic short leg, ruling out of a physiologic (functional) short leg, and appropriate measures to relieve the stress caused by it.

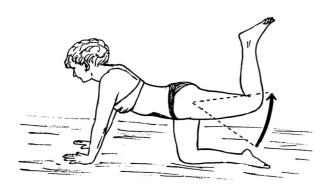

Figure 6–6 Gluteus maximus exercise.

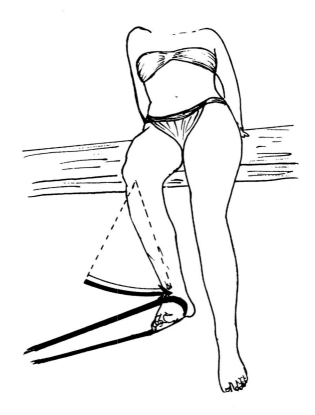

Figure 6–7 Piriformis muscle exercise.

Passive Hyperextension of the Knee

Passive hyperextension is not to be mistaken for genu recurvatum, where the knee (usually both knees) is congenitally hyperextended.

To test for passive hyperextension, grasp both heels and elevate them from the table, keeping them even (Figure 6–8A). Observe the knees for the ability to relax into the position. Edema is possible if the knee bounces back to flexion and if the screw-home movement does not occur.

If no bouncing back is present, allow the legs to remain suspended. If this is not painful, ask the patient to try to relax the leg muscles further. Shake the legs gently to check if the patient has relaxed them. This provides an opportunity to compare both legs thoroughly and may provide invaluable signs for investigation.

With the muscles consciously relaxed, a comparison of the true bulk of the muscles is possible. Look for obvious muscle contractions, differences in size, the dimpling usually found medial and superior to the patella (if absent, a sign of edema), and atrophy (usually of the VMO).

If one knee is hyperextended more than the other, gently press down on each knee, not only feeling for reaction but observing as well (Figure 6–8B). If the affected knee is hyperextended, the popliteus muscle must allow it. The popliteus

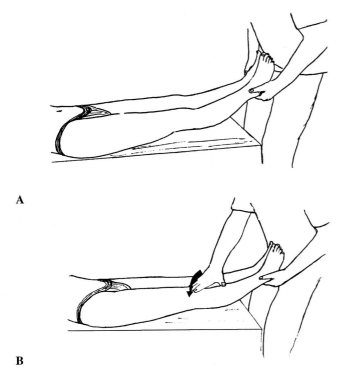

A

B

Figure 6–8 (**A** and **B**) Test for passive hyperextension.

muscle initiates flexion of the knee from hyperextension to the beginning of flexion, where the hamstring muscles participate.

The seemingly normal knee may be a genu recurvatum that cannot hyperextend because of edema. Normal hyperextension is 5° to 10°.

Laterally Rotated Femur and Knee Problems

Any problem that produces a laterally rotated femur makes it necessary to walk with the foot deviated laterally (Figure 6–9). This produces strain on the foot, causing pronation (Figure 6–10) as well as strain of the medial structures of the knee. Not only does this place strain on the medial ligamental structures of the knee, but it also strains the popliteus and the vastus medialis muscles.

Laterally rotated femur may occur from the following:

- hypertonic piriformis and/or gluteus maximus muscles (common in minor slip-fall injuries)
- strained or stretched medial rotators of the femur (anterior fibers of the gluteus minimus and medius and the tensor fascia lata)
- change of habit pattern to avoid pain of an iliopectineal bursitis
- exercise programs that simulate the lotus position in yoga

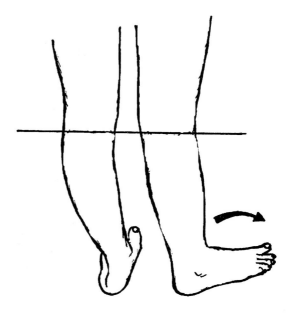

Figure 6–9 Lateral rotation.

- sitting on the foot (a position assumed by individuals, especially women, with short legs that do not reach the floor in a normal chair)
- sitting with one ankle over the opposite knee

The most common cause is sleeping in the prone position, in which the feet must be turned one way or the other. If turned to the right, the right knee must be flexed, which coupled with the turning of the foot produces the laterally rotated femur. The head must be turned toward the same side as the feet. Thus the prone sleeper usually has an imbalance not only of the hip

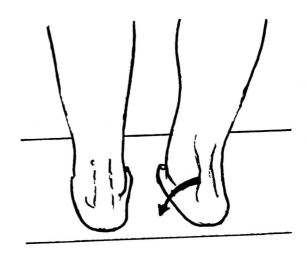

Figure 6–10 Pronated right foot.

and knee but of the cervical-thoracic junction as well.[1] It is necessary to treat the knee problem, but it is also necessary to break the sleep habit as well or the problem just keeps repeating itself.

A sleep habit cannot be altered on the conscious level. The patient may alter the position upon going to sleep, but as soon as deep sleep occurs the prone position will be assumed. Three methods of breaking the sleep habit have been found successful:

1. Tape table tennis balls on each side of the abdomen, 2 to 3 in from the umbilicus. This provides an irritant upon rolling over, disturbing not only sleep but the sleep habit. This method usually takes three to four sleep-disturbed nights to break the habit.

2. Also requiring three to four nights to break the habit is the method of tying a belt around the knees, securing them together. Use a small, soft pillow between the knees to prevent pelvic torque. This makes it possible to sleep supine or on the side but impossible to sleep prone.

3. Use an extremely large pillow next to the body to prevent rolling over during sleep. Place the pillow on the side away from the edge of the mattress. This method works for some individuals, but it is not as effective as the first two.

No matter how severe the knee problem, postural stresses as noted above must be taken into consideration. If postural stresses are considered the primary cause of symptoms, treatment should be directed to include their correction. If postural stress is present in the trauma case, corrective treatment should be included at the earliest possible time.

Pronated Foot and Knee Problems

Pronation of the foot (see Figure 6–10) places valgus strain on the knee.[2,3] If pronation of one or both feet is present, a determination must be made as to whether the pronation is the result of other postural strains. If so, these should be addressed. The pronation may also be a local problem due to injury, worn-out shoes, or habit patterns.

Treatment may include exercises for the anterior and posterior tibialis muscles to elevate the arch, the use of orthotics if exercises fail, alteration of poor habit patterns, and throwing away of worn-out shoes.

Use of Orthotics

There are many types of orthotics in use today, including hard materials, soft pliable materials, and plastic. Some are reinforced with metal and leather. There are many ways of determining what shape the orthotic should be, including:

- weight bearing onto a Styrofoam form, which is then sent away to a technician, who manufactures the orthotic
- weight bearing using an inked tape to produce the imprint of the plantar surface of the foot, which again is sent away for manufacturing
- production of a non-weight-bearing cast, again sent for manufacturing
- use of any of the above with the practitioner manufacturing his or her own orthotic from whatever materials he or she desires.

Each of the above methods (and there are others) claims its share of success.

Theories abound as to when to apply orthotics, either at the beginning of treatment or after other treatment has failed. In the author's opinion, the only time an orthotic should be used at the beginning of treatment is when the symptoms are caused by trauma and ligamental damage is suspected to have occurred. To apply an orthotic without first trying conservative care only provides a crutch for the foot, forever. It may correct the distortion immediately, but it does not correct the condition that caused it. Therefore, orthotics should be used only after exercises and correction of the postural causes have been tried.

KNEE DYSFUNCTION DUE TO ORGANIC PROBLEMS

Gallbladder

If the patient displays a hyperextended knee during the examination in the erect posture and it is verified by hyperextension in the supine position, test the popliteus muscle.

To test the popliteus, flex the knee to approximately 120°, diminishing the medial hamstring support (Figure 6–11A). Place the foot in medial rotation, and instruct the patient to hold it there. Do not have the patient medially rotate the foot (patients often will medially rotate *and* invert the foot, bringing into play the anterior tibialis muscle). With the patient holding, attempt lateral rotation of the foot while supporting the heel (Figure 6–11B). Do not use the toes for a contact; use a broad contact.

If the popliteus muscle tests weak, the possibility of a problem in the gallbladder should be investigated (see Appendix A). Inquire as to whether any gallbladder symptoms are present (eg, flatulence, heartburn, upper right quadrant pain, and/or constipation).

Palpate T4–5 for fixation. Palpate just below the right costal cartilage and the paraspinal muscles of T4–5 for tenderness and tension. If the popliteus muscle is weak and a fixation at T4–5 is present, adjust the fixation and retest the muscle. If the muscle responds yet both symptoms reappear on subsequent visits, investigation into gallbladder dysfunction is necessary.

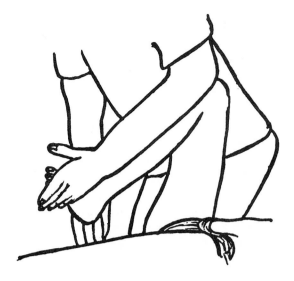

A

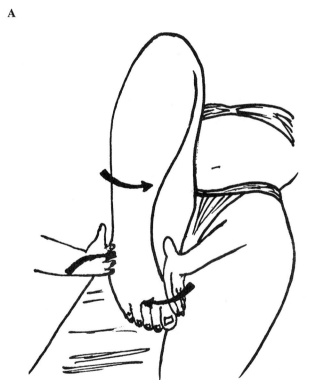

B

Figure 6–11 (A) Contacts to test the popliteus muscle. (B) Popliteus muscle test.

Duodenum

If a weak quadriceps femoris (QF) muscle is present that does not respond to manual assistance, adjust all fixations that may affect function of the QF. Consider the possibility of duodenum dysfunction if the lack of response is not caused by

pain, if there are persistent fixations in the midthoracic spine, if there are tension and tenderness of the paraspinal muscles of T7–11 and tenderness and tension just above the umbilicus, and if digestive symptoms are present (see Appendix A).

STRAINS

Dorland's Illustrated Medical Dictionary defines strain as follows: to overexercise; to use to an extreme and harmful degree; or an overstretching or overexertion of some part of the musculature. Cailliet[4(p.63)] defines strain as "the physical force imposed upon the ligamentous tissues possibly exceeding normal stress but not causing deformation or damage to the tissues. Physiological recovery is expected." For the purposes of this text, strain refers to injuries to the musculature only and may be classified as follows:

1. *mild*—stress or injury to the musculature that interferes with normal function but with little or no fiber damage
2. *moderate*—injury to the musculature sufficient to prevent muscle function without pain; palpable areas of pain and/or edema within the muscle, the origin, or the insertion; some fiber damage, yet the muscle may function in spite of the pain
3. *severe*—tearing of a major portion of the muscle fibers, preventing use of the muscle.

Mild Strain

Examination

During the examination, posture may be found to be altered as a result of malfunction. A mild strain may produce a hypertonic reaction (eg, a "knuckle" in the deltoid). A muscle may not function up to par (eg, the popliteus muscle may be stretched after sitting with the legs suspended and the feet on a stool, allowing hyperextension). Testing of the muscle may cause cheating by the patient, that is, shifting to allow recruitment of other muscles to respond to the command. Testing of the muscle may be nearly normal, yet the muscle may shake during the test.

Palpation of the muscles is important. Areas of hypertonic muscle fibers or lack of muscle tone may be detected only on palpation. Without careful palpation, many strains may be overlooked simply because the muscle tested nearly normal. If the areas are left untreated, altered patterns of function could lead to more problems in the future.

In the study of muscles and their function, the tendency often is to assume that if the muscle tests nearly normal no damage has occurred. Many of the larger muscles of the body that originate or insert over a large area may test 100%, with the bulk of the muscle providing the resistance. A smaller portion of the muscle, however, may be functioning at only 50%.

A good example of this is the gluteus maximus muscle with origins on the ilia, sacrum, and coccyx and the insertion into a long area on the posterolateral femur. It may test normal even though the coccygeal fibers are strained because the bulk of the muscle is normal.

Treatment Modalities

Many modalities and techniques are available for use by the practitioner.

Ultrasound. Ultrasound has been used for many years for its high-frequency sound waves to produce a deep massage and heat. The author uses ultrasound over an entrapped medial meniscus after the adjustment has been made.

Friction Massage. The operator's fingers are applied directly on the skin over the tissue without lubrication. The massage is directed across the tendon, with the operator's contact not moving on the patient's skin. Deep friction is applied to the patient's tolerance. This of course is painful and, in the author's opinion, questionable in its results.

Goading of the Origin and/or Insertion of a Ligament. This is similar to the friction massage, but application is directed over the origin or insertion of the ligament. Again, theories abound as to why this technique works, sometimes. The author has used this technique where mild ligamental strain or possible mild periosteal separation was suspected. It is not the treatment of choice, but it may be used as a last resort.

Goading of the Origin and/or Insertion of a Muscle. Again, this is similar to friction massage but is directed over the origin or insertion of a muscle suspected of injury. The author finds this technique useful for several reasons:

- In the beginning it requires that the practitioner learn *where* the origin and insertion are (an excellent learning opportunity).
- With knowledge of the origin and insertion as well as common sense, the practitioner will gain a better understanding of the function of the affected muscle.
- With a mild strain, goading of the origin and insertion often will cause an immediate response. Many times this becomes a diagnostic sign and also indicates the severity of the injury.

Electrical Stimulation. Electrical stimulation may be used in cases of muscle disuse. Contractions may be induced without effort on the part of the patient and without movement of the joint involved, if called for.

Cryotherapy. Cold therapy is used in many forms and includes ice massage, use of fluoromethane spray, and use of ice packs. If has been shown that the application of cold therapy for 10 minutes on and 10 minutes off three times causes the cold temperature to remain in the tissue longer than with 20-minute applications.

The author prefers to use the following technique, especially on the extremities:

1. Fold two towels to the size desired.
2. Wet and ring them out so that they do not drip.
3. Place in the freezer for 1 hour or until they freeze.
4. Place directly on the skin or over the taped surface.

The surface of a frozen towel will start to thaw immediately, thus preventing ice burn. By changing the towels, applications may be made as necessary.

Heat. One of the common errors made by patients is the application of a heating pad to a place that hurts. Patients report, "I started hurting on Friday, so I used the heating pad, and it felt better. It got worse, though, and last night I laid on the heating pad all night for relief. Today, I can barely walk."

The application of topical heat, especially with a heating pad, only brings circulation to the tissue. The blood vascular system continues its flow, but the lymphatics, which depend on motion, only become more congested. This allows the toxins normally carried away by the lymphatics to remain in the local tissue. Therefore, when the patient is off the pad for a while, whatever relief was gained from the pad disappears, and the condition is now worse.

The author prefers the following treatment:

1. Fold a towel to the desired size.
2. Wet and ring it out so that it does not drip.
3. Place in the microwave oven for 2 to 3 minutes, depending on the oven. *Caution*: Be sure to check the inside of the towel before using. Often the towel seems to keep on cooking and will be too hot.
4. With the knee elevated higher than the hip, apply the hot towel over the affected knee *for no more than 2 minutes.*
5. Remove the towel and place it back in the microwave to reheat.
6. Move the joint gently through as much of the normal range of motion as possible for approximately 2 minutes.
7. Repeat the process five to six times.

Theoretically, the application of moist heat brings increased circulation to the area involved. If allowed to continue for more than 2 minutes, however, the lymphatics become overloaded. By removal of the moist heat followed by movement of the joint, the lymphatics are drained, and the process may be repeated as needed.

Treatment of Specific Conditions

If severe damage to the knee structures has been eliminated and only a mild strain has occurred, treatment should be directed toward eliminating postural stresses, if present, and stretching hypertonic muscles or portions thereof.

Vastus Lateralis. Careful palpation may reveal a hypertonic vastus lateralis muscle with a tight iliotibial tract. This condition often accompanies weakened VMO. In extreme cases, surgical intervention has been used to release the pull on the patella laterally. This of course should be the last resort. Correction may be accomplished by instituting an exercise program for the weakened VMO and stretching of the vastus lateralis muscle.

To stretch the vastus lateralis, flex the knee to 90° and, using both thumbs, apply steady pressure to stretch the fibers palpated as hypertonic (usually the lower third of the muscle).

Stretching for 30 to 45 seconds of a hypertonic muscle that has resulted from an opposing weakened muscle may relieve some pain and allow improved function. This can at best be only temporary, however, and can only serve as a method of relief until exercises can take effect.

If examination reveals that the muscle is hypertonic as a result of trauma, use heavy digital pressure over the tight area to relax the tissues. Manually stretch the muscle, and then apply moist heat for 2 to 3 minutes. Move the muscle gently, allowing it to move from partial contraction to its full length three to four times. Restretch manually, and repeat the moist heat and movement. Instruct the patient to repeat the moist heat and movement at home five times per session for three to four sessions in 24 hours. Finally, reevaluate.

Quadriceps Femoris. In the elderly patient, in whom bending, squatting, and other activities involving extreme knee flexion are no longer performed, a shortened QF is not unusual. Elderly patients who have been treated with cortisone injections for knee symptoms must be suspected of having this condition.

Treatment may be instituted immediately by applying steady pressure inferiorly on the patella to stretch the QF overall (Figure 6–12). This may be followed by stretching of the individual fibers if needed.

The patient may stretch the QF by lying on a table, couch, or bed with the affected limb off to the side. The patient hyperflexes the knee and extends the hip by holding the foot (Figure 6–13). Where possible, the same principle may be applied while standing. To increase the tension, have the patient posteriorly rotate the pelvis by using the abdominal muscles (Figure 6–14). Either method must be repeated several times every day until the full range of motion is restored.

Hamstrings. Normally the hamstring muscles do not come into play until the hip is flexed to 30°. If the hamstring muscles are hypertonic or shortened, instruction for the patient at home should include either of the following methods of stretching with applications of moist heat before and after.

Place the foot of the affected limb on a chair, keep the knee extended, and lean forward. *Do not move around*; simply

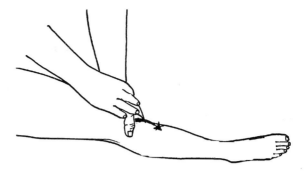

Figure 6–12 QF stretch.

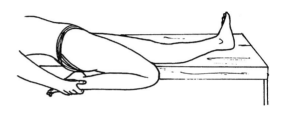

Figure 6–13 Supine QF stretch.

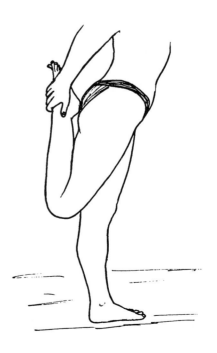

Figure 6–14 Standing QF stretch.

stretch and hold until a release is felt, then slowly relax from the position. Do not stretch hard enough to cause pain.

The better method is to sit on the floor with the pelvis and back securely against the wall. Place the heel on a stool. Using the hand, apply pressure to straighten the knee (Figure 6–15).

Triceps Surae (Gastrocnemius and Soleus) and Plantaris. Shortened triceps surae and plantaris muscles are a common problem that may produce symptoms in the foot and knee and, in turn, problems in the function of the pelvis and spine.

The gastrocnemius muscle is the largest muscle producing plantar flexion and the only one of significance to cross the knee (the plantaris is small and sometimes absent). The soleus, posterior tibialis, flexor hallucis longus, and peroneus longus all contribute to plantar flexion of the foot without any direct influence on knee function.

If these muscles are shortened, the range of motion will be limited in dorsiflexion. Often the patient cannot dorsiflex past 90° (Figure 6–16).

In the normal stride, the hindfoot remains on the surface until the ankle flexes well past 90° before pushing off, allowing the body to travel forward (Figure 6–17). With a shortened gastrocnemius muscle, as the leg approaches the 90° position the patient shortens the stride on the opposite limb, giving a mincing step. Alternatively, when the leg reaches 90° the body weight is thrust directly on the metatarsals to push off (rather than the normal transfer of weight through the foot as a whole; Figure 6–18).

Attempted stretching by the examiner is usually futile. If the muscle is shortened, it requires stretching over 2 to 3 weeks to restore to normal.

Patients may be instructed in several methods of stretching. While striding forward on the opposite limb, keep the knee straight, and apply pressure to attempt to place the heel on the floor (Figure 6–19). While sitting with the leg extended, use a belt or tubing to pull the foot into dorsiflexion and hold (Figure 6–20). The best method the author has found is with the use of a small slant board (13 × 13 in, rising to 5½ in from the floor in the front). By placing the board in a convenient location, the patient may stand on it many times during the day

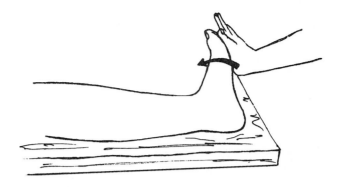

Figure 6–16 Limited ankle dorsiflexion.

(with the patient who cannot flex past 90°, standing on the board without holding onto something is not possible). By standing on the board for 3 to 4 minutes several times per day, dorsiflexion increases rapidly (Figure 6–21).

Restoration to Normal Function of the Weakened, Strained, or Stretched Muscle

Quadriceps Femoris. The VMO is the most common muscle fiber affected in both traumatic and nontraumatic cases seen in the office.

If the QF tests weak with or without pain, retest with support. Hook a thumb over the patella with the fingers toward the origin of the VMO. Secure the patella medially and proximally, and retest. If the fulcrum of the QF is diminished because of lax VMO fibers only, the muscle will test nearly normal[1] (Figures 6–22 and 6–23).

In the case of a mild strain, goading of the origin of the VMO, causing it to contract, is sufficient to allow retesting without manual assistance, and the QF may test normal. If so,

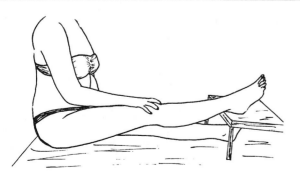

Figure 6–15 Hamstring muscle stretch.

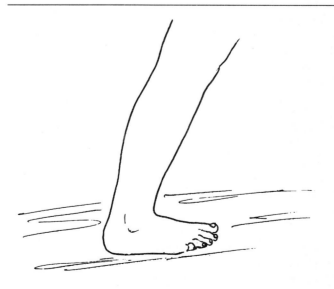

Figure 6–17 Normal ankle during stride.

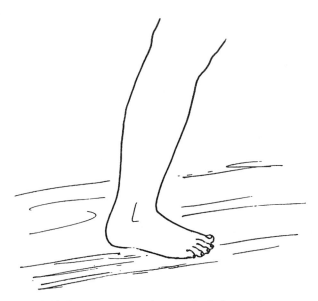

Figure 6–18 Short gastrocnemius muscle during stride.

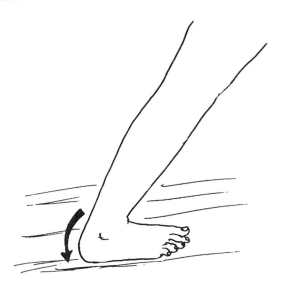

Figure 6–19 Gastrocnemius stretch.

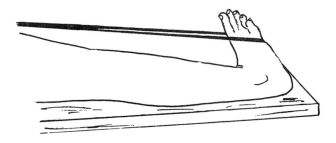

Figure 6–20 Gastrocnemius stretch with belt or tubing.

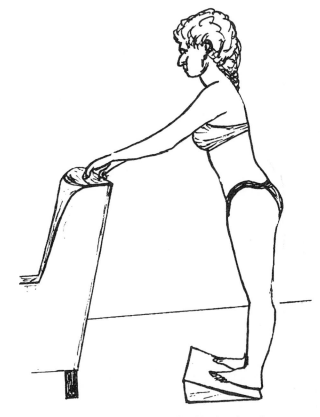

Figure 6–21 Gastrocnemius stretch with slant board.

mild exercises should be all that are necessary to restore function to normal.

If the QF responds with manual assistance but after goading fails to respond, it would indicate that the muscle fibers have been stretched and weakened over a long time and need exercise or that it is in fact a moderate strain with some fibers torn and needs rest, support (see taping under moderate strain, below), and then exercise.

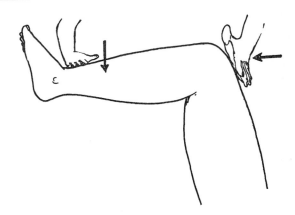

Figure 6–22 QF muscle test.

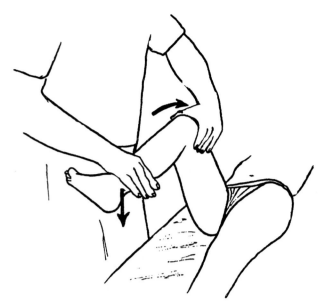

Figure 6–23 QF muscle test with patellar support.

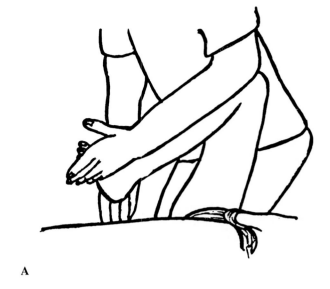

A

If the QF fails to respond with manual assistance, recheck for fixations of the knee, for fixations of the lumbosacral spine, and for pain upon pressure in the trochlear groove. Recheck the other QF muscles and, if suspicious, manually assist them and check again. Recheck for, and correct, fixations found in T7–11. If there is no response, manually assist the VMO and retest (in case both problems are present). Without pain on testing and with failure to respond to manual assistance, palpate just above the umbilicus for a reflex from the duodenum. If fixations were found at T7–11, investigation into possible duodenal problems should be done.

Popliteus Muscle. Test the popliteus muscle with the knee flexed to at least 100° to eliminate medial hamstring involvement (see Figure 6–24, A and B). If weak, goad the insertion on the tibia (see Figure 6–25).

Retest after goading. If the response is nearly normal, gentle exercises to restore function may be all that are necessary. If the popliteus muscle fails to respond, recheck for fixations of the knee, for lumbosacral fixations, and for fixations at T4–5 (if present, adjust and retest). If the muscle responds, inquire as to whether any gallbladder symptoms are present. If not, recheck at the next visit. If gallbladder symptoms are present or if muscle weakness *and* fixation at T4–5 are both present, on the next visit adjust the fixation and investigate the possibility of gallbladder dysfunction.

Sartorius and Gracilis. If either or both of these muscles test weak, repalpate for fixations of the knee, hip joint, pelvis, and lumbar spine.

Have the patient or an assistant hold the pelvis posteriorly and retest. If the muscle responds, the problem is with the support structure and should be treated accordingly.

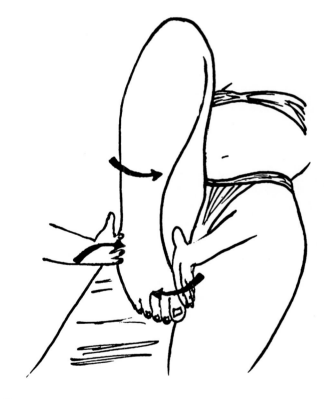

B

Figure 6–24 (A) Contacts to test the popliteus muscle. (B) Popliteus muscle test.

Goad the insertion at the pes anserinus. If the muscle responds, rest and mild exercise may be all that are necessary.

If the sartorius fails to respond, recheck for fixations at T8–10 and, if present, adjust. If the sartorius responds yet is

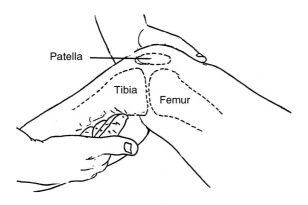

Figure 6–25 Goading the popliteus insertion.

weak on the next visit, and if the fixation is again present, the possibility of stress to the adrenal gland should be suspected (this is common in the menopausal patient, whether menopause is natural or surgically induced).

If the gracilis muscle fails to respond and the patient experienced an injury producing abduction and extension (eg, split-fall), carefully palpate the inferior ramus of the pubis and ischium for possible tears or periosteal separation (this is difficult to detect on the usual X-ray views and may require special views).

Hamstring Muscle. While testing the hamstrings, always maintain contact with the belly of the muscles in case a spasm occurs (Figures 6–26 and 6–27). If the muscle cramps, straighten the leg immediately and apply pressure on the belly of the muscle until the cramp ceases. Do no retest on this visit. The examiner must keep in mind that an upset in the calcium–phosphorus ratio or a vitamin E deficiency may lead to cramping.

If the hamstrings test weak, recheck for fixations of the lumbosacral spine and for fixations of the hip and knee joints. Repalpate the entire muscle for possible tears. Palpate the ischial tuberosity for possible bursitis, periosteal separation, or tendon tears. Palpate the plantaris muscle and, if palpable, goad gently for a few moments and then retest the hamstrings. The author has found that goading the plantaris muscle often produces a response when the hamstrings are retested. The plantaris muscle inserts some fibers into the flexor retinaculum that may somehow affect hamstring function. Finally, re-evaluate the popliteus muscle for weakness (which will interfere with function of the hamstrings).

If the medial hamstrings are suspected, carefully evaluate the sartorius and gracilis muscles, the insertion of the semimembranosus, and the pes anserinus for possible bursitis or muscle tear.

If the lateral hamstring is suspected, recheck the fibula for mobility (or lack of mobility) and all the muscles of the foot that originate on the fibula for dysfunction. Palpate the short

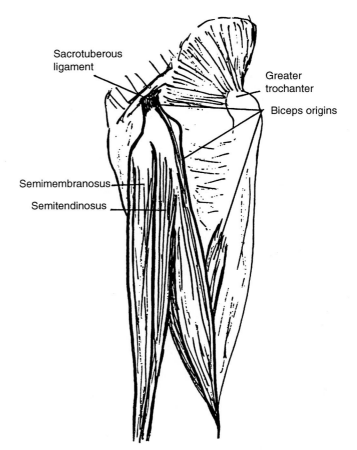

Figure 6–26 Right leg, posterior view showing hamstring muscles.

head of the biceps on the posterior femur for possible tears or areas of hypertonicity. If tone seems to be lacking, gently goad the origin. Palpate the fibula head insertion (behind the insertion and the lateral collateral ligament) for bursitis. Finally, recheck for pelvic fixations or instability.

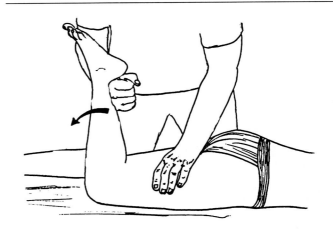

Figure 6–27 Hamstring muscle test.

Gastrocnemius Muscle. Seldom is the gastrocnemius muscle weak from a mild strain, but it is possible that a strain of one of the heads may lead to symptoms in the knee. Usually a unilateral strain of the head of the gastrocnemius muscle, especially the lateral head, produces foot symptoms. The patient may perform a toe-walk easily by recruiting the flexor hallucis longus. This alters the normal function of the foot and usually produces symptoms in the tarsals.

A mild strain that interferes with normal function yet reveals no severe damage to the tissues often provides the practitioner an opportunity to do more than just relieve the immediate problem. It may also allow correction of postural stress and habit patterns that could lead to severe degeneration later in life.

Moderate Strain

Injury to the musculature is often sufficient to prevent muscle function without pain and to produce palpable areas of pain and/or edema within the muscle, the tendon, the origin, or the insertion. A diagnosis of moderate strain would be considered if:

- no joint instability is found (it may be present with an instability and, if suspected, should be noted in the diagnosis; testing of the muscle is inconclusive in the presence of an instability, however)
- no joint edema is found
- muscle testing is not possible without pain, with or without manual support
- careful palpation reveals an area (or areas) of pain and/or edema within the muscle, tendon, origin, or insertion
- a muscle is stretched and elongated sufficiently to interfere with its normal function (this is included as a moderate strain even though no tears are suspected; elongation of a muscle over a long time requiring an exercise to strengthen *and* shorten the muscle usually requires support until the exercise program shows progress)

Treatment includes cessation of all activities that would place stress on the tissues involved. Adjust all fixations that might affect the area involved. Use ice therapy if edema is suspected (it will limit intramuscular bleeding if present). Support the musculature involved with tape or a brace. Correct any postural stresses that may be contributing to the problem.

After edema is reduced and/or after sufficient time has elapsed to allow repair of the tissues, mild exercises may be started with subsequent applications of moist heat for 2 to 3 minutes. If after exercise and moist heat application edema returns, cease the program and allow more time for tissue repair.

If a stretched, elongated muscle is involved, exercises may be performed immediately with support. There are many supports designed for the knee that are useful for assisting in instabilities. It has been the author's experience that the most effective means of supporting muscles of the knee is the use of elastic taping without an underwrap. Some individuals with light skin or with an allergy to adhesive tape, or individuals requiring long-term wearing of the support, may need a spray skin coating before taping.

Oblique Fibers of the Vastus Medialis

If the QF tests weak and responds to manual support (see Figures 6–22 and 6–23), goad the origin of the VMO. If the muscle fails to respond and cannot perform adequately, taping is usually necessary. Taping provides support of the muscle, allowing the patient to be ambulatory with less, or no, pain.

With the patient supine, rest the leg over the operator's thigh only slightly flexed. Begin the first tape well below the knee for secure attachment. Traverse the patella with the tape, following the direction of the VMO. Extend the tape around the thigh as far as the vastus lateralis muscle (Figure 6–28).

Apply the second tape slightly lateral to the first, traversing the patella and following the direction of the lowest fibers of the VMO (Figure 6–29). Apply the third tape at a slightly different angle and follow the highest fibers of the VMO (Figure 6–30).

Apply two or three strips along the medial leg for additional support of the medial knee structures (Figure 6–31). The adductor, sartorius, gracilis, and semitendinosus muscles may be involved. Secure the ends of the tape both proximally and distally to prevent rolling up and to provide more security (Figure 6–32).

Retest the quadriceps without manual support. If the muscle responded before with manual support and the tape is now applied properly, the QF should respond as well with the tape on (Figure 6–33).

Taping may only be needed for 3 to 4 days, and if upon reevaluation function is restored the tape may be removed. In the more severe of the moderate strain cases, it may be neces-

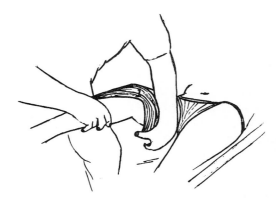

Figure 6–28 VMO support, first tape.

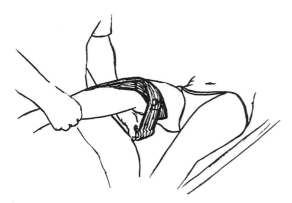

Figure 6–29 VMO support, second tape.

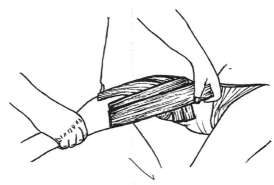

Figure 6–31 Taping for additional support of medial knee structures.

sary to leave the tape on for 7 to 10 days, depending upon patient cooperation with the exercise program. If so, the tape may have to be reinforced after 3 or 4 days of wear.

Vastus Lateralis

Although relatively rare, a blow to the medial side of the knee may cause damage to the vastus lateralis and possible iliotibial tract strain. It is extremely rare that the vastus lateralis would be strained in a postural fault. If a vastus lateralis strain should occur, taping is the reverse of that for the VMO.

Popliteus

Popliteus muscle strain is common in ski injuries involving lateral rotation of the foot with the knee bent (Figure 6–34). The momentum produces damage to the medial knee structures and to the VMO as well. Taping of the popliteus may be included in taping of the VMO.

Begin taping on the medial leg, well below the knee. Follow the direction of the popliteal fibers as low as possible on the lateral condyle of the femur. Continue taping until sufficient surface is covered to support the muscle (Figure 6–35).

Apply a second tape more posteriorly and following the muscle fibers, ending up proximal to the first. Apply addi-

tional tapes if necessary along the same track (Figure 6–36). Secure the ends (Figure 6–37).

Sartorius and Gracilis

Strains of the sartorius and gracilis are usually associated with VMO or popliteus muscle strains, and, if suspected, additional tape may be applied supporting the pes anserinus area and extending up the medial thigh.

Medial Hamstring

If the damage occurred at the insertion of the semitendinosus with the sartorius, gracilis, and popliteus, additional tape may be applied following the muscle up the thigh.

If damage to the semimembranosus is suspected, adequate taping is not possible directly on the insertion. The knee should be secured in a flexed position and rested until the tissue mends.

If both hamstrings are strained involving fibers other than the insertion, taping of the entire posterior aspect of the thigh to prevent full extension of the knee may be necessary.

Lateral Hamstring

If fibers of the biceps femoris other than those at or near the insertion are torn, taping the entire posterior thigh may be necessary and should include the insertion described below.

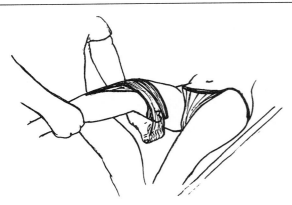

Figure 6–30 VMO support, third tape.

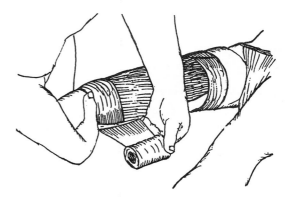

Figure 6–32 VMO support, securing the tape ends.

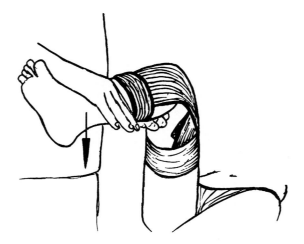

Figure 6–33 QF test with tape support.

Before taping for an injury involving the biceps insertion, motion palpate the fibula head. If damage has occurred to the muscles opposing the biceps as well, taping should include the fibula.

With the knee flexed at 10° to 15°, start the tape 6 in below the fibula head, and use three to four strips of tape along the route of the fibers to approximately halfway up the thigh. Secure both ends of the tape.

Summary

One of the problems in practice is patient control. The patient who has experienced pain, has had support on for some time, and reaches the point in the treatment program where the support may be removed is vulnerable. If the patient is careful and continues the exercise program, there is no problem. It is necessary to explain to the patient, however, that he or she has

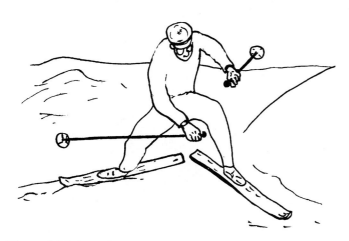

Figure 6–34 Common mechanism of popliteus muscle strain.

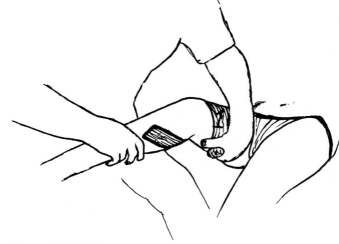

Figure 6–35 Popliteus support, first tape.

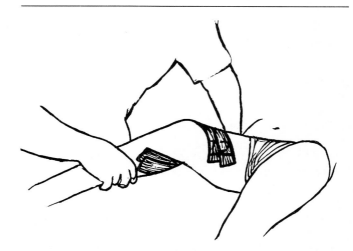

Figure 6–36 Popliteus support, second tape.

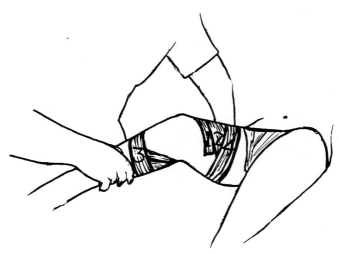

Figure 6–37 Popliteus support, securing the tape ends.

now reached a level that is precarious. With care, some normal function may be resumed, and exercise is now more important than it was at the beginning of the treatment program. Patients should be warned that the joint structure is now highly susceptible to reinjury that will undo all the progress attained so far.

Severe Strain

Severe strain involves tearing of a major portion of a muscle, tendon, or periosteal attachment.

Quadriceps Mechanism

Tears may occur in the following locations:

- within the muscle itself (muscle tears from direct trauma while the muscle is contracted may occur at the point of impact)
- at the muscle-tendon junction (this is the most common location)
- at the upper attachment of the tendon on the patella
- at the lower attachment of the tendon on the patella
- within the patella tendon itself
- at the attachment of the tendon on the tibia tubercle

Tears at the muscle-tendon junction occur in the athlete during abrupt deceleration as the foot strikes with the knee flexed and/or as a result of direct trauma. In the aged person who is not in good physical condition, tearing may occur with relatively minor incidents, such as stepping off the curb unexpectedly.

Ambulation is not possible. Pain is immediate and excruciating with forced flexion or attempted extension. Careful palpation reveals a depression in the muscle.

Treatment involves immobilization by splint in full extension with ice. The use of anti-inflammatory agents may be necessary, requiring medical consultation. If the tear is extensive enough to require surgery, the patient should be referred to a competent surgeon who will cooperate for the patient's benefit and allow rehabilitation under chiropractic care. Surgery, if necessary, is not possible at the early stage and, if performed, will probably fail.

If the injury is not extensive, conservative care may include adjusting all fixations that may relate to the lower extremity. As soon as the edema is reduced, mild stretching and moist heat should be applied to prevent excessive scar tissue formation and fixation of the muscles. If edema stays reduced, the use of alternating ice and heat is useful. When full range of motion is possible, mild exercises may be started and increased to restore normal function of the QF. Reevaluation of the comparative strength and coordination of both lower extremities is necessary to remove habit patterns formed as a result of the disability.

Tears of the tendon attachments to the patella, the tibial tubercle, or within the tendon itself occur more often in the eld-

erly patient, especially those who may have some degree of degeneration of the tendon, the bone structure, or both. The elderly patient may stumble while walking down stairs or stepping off a curb unexpectedly. He or she will experience instant pain and will collapse, unable to bear weight on the limb.

If the tear occurs at the superior patellar attachment, the patella may palpate as a low patella. If so, an interruption may be palpated. Radiographs will reveal a fragment superior to the patella if it is an avulsion.

If the tear occurs at the inferior border, the patella will appear high with a contracted QF and a palpable interruption in the tendon. If it is avulsed, radiographs will reveal a fragment below the patella.

Avulsion of the patellar tendon form the tibia tubercle occurs in the young (see discussion of Osgood-Schlatter disease) and in the elderly. Tendon tears and avulsions sufficient to require surgery should be referred immediately to prevent complications that will make repair more difficult.

Patellar Dislocation

Normal function of the patellar-femoral articulation is dependent on normal alignment of the knee (Q angle), the QF mechanism, and the shape of the bone structures[5-7] (Figure 6–38).

During full extension, the patella rests on a fat pad superior to the trochlear groove and is maintained in position only by fasciae and the action of the muscles. As flexion begins, the facets of the patella articulate with the medial and lateral sides of the trochlear groove between the femur condyles. The lateral condyle of the femur projects farther anteriorly than medially, providing a barrier to assist in retaining the patella in the groove through full flexion[6,8] (Figure 6–39).

During flexion, the patella progressively articulates further inferiorly on the femur. Smooth movement during flexion, with the patella retained in the neutral position, is maintained by action of the QF muscles. The VMO provides the strength to hold the patella medially against the pressures exerted through the Q angle (Figure 6–40).

A comparison may be made of the two walls of the trochlear groove during examination (Figures 6–41 and 6–42).

Patellar dislocation has the following possible etiologies:

- congenital malformation
- trauma
- valgus knee
- weak VMO
- lack of anterior projection of the lateral femur condyle
- shallow trochlear groove (may be the result of lack of anterior projection of the lateral femur condyle)
- anomalous patella
- elongated patellar ligament with patella alta (elevated patella)

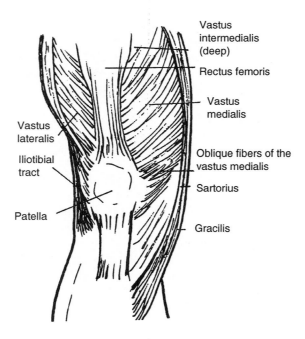

Figure 6–38 Right knee, anterior view.

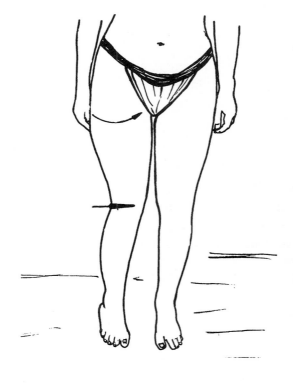

Figure 6–40 Valgus knee and medially rotated femur (increased Q angle).

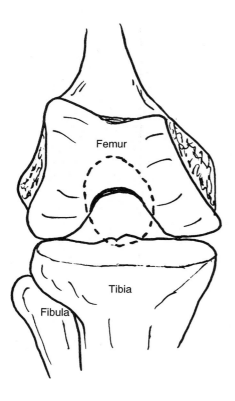

Figure 6–39 Right knee, flexed showing the distal end of the femur.

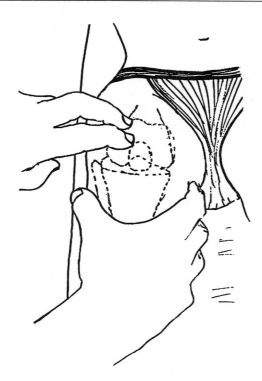

Figure 6–41 Palpation of the lateral trochlear wall.

- anomalous lateral attachment of the patellar ligament on the tibia tubercle.

Congenital. Anomalous patella, lateral condyle, and lateral insertion of the patellar ligament may make it necessary for surgical intervention in the infant. These are usually associated with a valgus knee and extreme lateral rotation of the tibia.

Examination of the infant should include careful palpation of the lower extremity for valgus knee, lateral rotation of the tibia, and position of the patella. Although dislocation may not occur, the malfunction should not be allowed to continue. Any malfunction may provide the ingredients for problems at the beginning of ambulation.

A laterally displaced patella in the child produces weakness of knee function and abnormal foot, hip, pelvis, and back function. It may also cause a wearing away of the lateral condyle (if normal to start with), which may later lead to patellar dislocation.

Traumatic. Dislocation due to trauma usually occurs with the knee extended with lateral torque applied, such as in swinging a bat.[6] With the leg extended, the patella is superior to the trochlear groove and dependent on the muscles and fasciae to hold it in place.

If dislocation occurs, replacement may be accomplished by extending the knee and flexing the hip, removing some of the tension from the rectus femoris muscle.

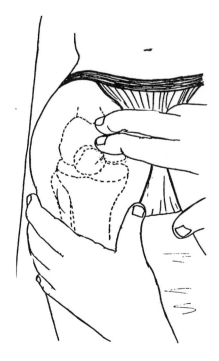

Figure 6–42 Palpation of the medial trochlear wall.

Once dislocation has occurred, the possibility of its recurring is great unless the predisposing factors are corrected.

Treatment. In the infant, manipulation of the knee and all fixations that may affect the knee is necessary. Correction of muscle malfunction and/or overdevelopment of muscles to offset anomalous bone structure takes on a whole new meaning in infants and children and requires patience and cooperative parents.

In the infant with a medially rotated femur, frequent play by tickling (goading) the insertion of the piriformis and gluteus maximus muscles may stimulate function. Frequent goading may alter an infant's habit patterns in a short time. The same procedure may be used at the origin of the VMO and the popliteus muscle.

With the child who is ambulatory, the same procedure may be applied. With some thought, games may be used to provoke exercise of the muscles involved.

Once the child is old enough, correction of any rotational problem of the lower extremity is helped greatly by use of roller skates. The child may have to be pulled at first by the parents until he or she is old enough to skate on his or her own. Skating is excellent training to correct either a lateral or a medial rotation.

When the child reaches an age where cooperation in an exercise program is expected, muscle development is limited only by the diligence of the child and parents.

In adults, treatment should be directed toward correction of any and all postural stresses and muscle weaknesses that predispose to lateral movement of the patella. If a bone anomaly is present or if the muscle fibers and fasciae have been torn or stretched, overdevelopment of the muscles is necessary to give sufficient stability to the knee.

Case Study. The following case history is an example of this approach. A 30-year-old woman who was unable to perform a squat ever to her memory presented with a history of constant pain in both knees for 8 years and weakness and occasional pain before that. Radiographs revealed underdeveloped or worn away lateral femur condyles bilaterally (probably congenital); the condition of the right one was more extreme. A photograph of the patient at 8 years of age seated on a bench showed both patellae deviated extremely laterally.

Surgical intervention had been proposed by several orthopedic surgeons, which would require two to three surgeries on each knee and had only a low probability of success.

Examination revealed the following:

- patient apprehension with any lateral pressure on the patella
- extremely weak QF on testing
- QF response to manual assistance
- minimal valgus knee (further evidence of congenital malformation)
- no medial rotation of the femur

- weakness of the popliteus muscle upon testing
- on palpation, practically nonexistent lateral wall of the trochlear groove (painful to the touch)
- extremely tight iliotibial tract and vastus lateralis
- VMO with little bulk and only minimal muscle tone on palpation

An attempt to squat with assistance from the author and an associated failed with pain at approximately 20° of flexion.

Treatment involved taping of the knee for popliteus and VMO support and medial stress. An undercoating was used because of the expected long duration of wear. The foot, knee, and pelvis were adjusted, as were fixations of the spine. Exercises for the VMO and popliteus muscles using tubing were devised that could be performed at home and in her office.

With the tape applied, the patient reported that she felt more secure and that walking produced only 10% of the pain she had experienced before. An attempt to squat with the tape on failed at 20° to 25°.

After 2 weeks of tape support and exercise, the patient was able to squat with the tape on, balancing herself with hand contact that bore part of the weight. Return to standing was not possible.

After 4 weeks of support, adjustment of the affected structures, and diligent exercise, the patient was able to do a squat and to return to standing with the tape on. Removal of the tape revealed an improved QF, but squatting could not be performed with the tape off.

Six weeks after the initiation of treatment, the patient presented with greatly improved strength upon testing of the VMO and popliteus without manual or tape support. Squatting without the tape support was still not possible, but some progress was seen. The tape was removed.

Eight weeks found the patient able to squat with minimal assistance (mostly balancing). Four months after onset of treatment, the patient could perform a complete squat and return to erect posture without pain, restriction, or great difficulty. Upon final examination and release from treatment, the patient exhibited a VMO the size of that of a male bodybuilder with overdevelopment sufficient to overcome the lateral condyle deficit. Even though the overdevelopment was undesirable cosmetically, it was far superior to the scars from surgeries that had little chance for success.

Summary. A treatment program can only be successful with a cooperative and determined patient. By providing a proper examination and informing the patient of what is to be expected, even the most difficult patient has a good chance to succeed.

TENDINITIS AND OVERUSE PROBLEMS

Inflammation and irritation of the tendons, their attachments, and the adjacent tissues may be caused by long-distance running, repetitive activities, and postural deficiencies such as pronated feet or increased Q angle. Careful palpation of the tissues around the knee is essential for establishing a correct diagnosis.

Iliotibial Band Friction

The iliotibial band traverses across the lateral condyle of the femur during flexion (Figures 6–43 and 6–44). Inflammation may occur over the most prominent part of the lateral condyle as a result of excessive friction. Abnormal movement of the iliotibial band over the condyle during activity may be the cause of friction.[6,7]

Symptoms of lateral knee pain sometimes extend to the front of the knee. Activities such as running or walking uphill and/or downhill may produce anterior knee symptoms. The patient may complain of symptoms in rising from sitting or lowering to sitting.

Although iliotibial band friction is common in long-distance runners, running itself is not the cause. Abnormal mechanics of the knee produces irritation. There are several causes of abnormal mechanics:

- increased Q angle
- weakened or stretched VMO
- pronated foot
- valgus knee
- varus knee

Each of the above may result in a hypertonic vastus lateralis muscle and possible tightness of the iliotibial band. Anatomic short leg is another possible cause of abnormal mechanics.

Diagnosis

Carefully palpate the lateral condyle while the patient flexes or extends the knee against resistance and varus stress. Pain on palpation may extend to the insertion on the anterior surface of the lateral tibial condyle.

Ober's test for a tight iliotibial tract may or may not be positive. If Ober's test is used as a diagnostic sign, it is important to secure the pelvis during the test. A weak quadratus lumborum muscle may allow the pelvis to move inferiorly, clouding the results (a weak quadratus lumborum muscle may be the cause of compensatory gluteus medius, gluteus minimus, and/or tensor fascia lata hypertonicity). In the author's opinion, Ober's test is for a short iliotibial tract and/or a short gluteus medius muscle. A short gluteus medius muscle (which occurs more often in men than in women) should not be confused with a short iliotibial tract.

Palpation of the iliotibial tract may reveal pain and excessive tightness. Some edema may be present at the site of friction on the lateral femur condyle and may extend to the insertion.

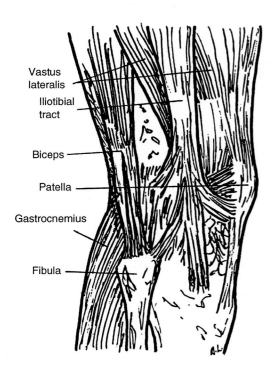

Vastus
lateralis

Iliotibial
tract

Biceps

Patella

Gastrocnemius

Fibula

Figure 6–43 Right knee, lateral view showing muscle attachments.

Careful palpation is necessary to eliminate or include other problems in the diagnosis. With the knee flexed to 30°, palpate the anterior knee joint line. Have the patient gently attempt knee extension. The first structure palpated moving posteriorly along the joint line is the iliotibial tract, which can now be traced to its insertion.

Treatment

Treatment comprises rest (complete cessation of the activities that produced the symptoms is necessary), ice to reduce edema and inflammation, and correction of the cause of dysfunction.

Adjust all fixations that could be related to the structures involved. Evaluate for an anatomic short leg. Eliminate the cause (or causes) of a medially or laterally rotated femur. Finally, evaluate for possible lateral tracking of the patella.

A weak quadratus lumborum muscle on the side of complaint may be the ultimate cause of a tight tract. Stretch the iliotibial tract.

Problems Involving the Biceps Femoris Tendon, Popliteus Tendon, and Lateral Collateral Ligament

Careful palpation is necessary to differentiate lateral collateral ligament, popliteus tendon, and biceps tendon problems.

The biceps tendon splits around the lateral collateral ligament in its attachment to the fibula head and sends fibers to

the ligament itself, the femoral condyle, and the fascia (Figure 6–45).

After locating the iliotibial tract as described above, with the knee in 30° of flexion, palpate from the anterior joint line, passing over the iliotibial tract (the first structure encountered). Have the patient relax the knee, and apply mild varus stress; the lateral collateral ligament becomes prominent.

Have the patient gently, laterally rotate the foot, and apply slight flexion to the knee; the biceps tendon is located easily because of its angle of insertion in flexion.

With the knee still in 30° of flexion, have the patient relax, gently medially rotate the foot, and then relax again several times. The activity makes it easy to palpate the popliteus origin (inferior and anterior to the femoral attachment of the lateral collateral ligament) and the tendon (posterior to the lateral collateral ligament as it crosses the joint line).

To treat problems of these tissues, adjust all structures involved or any that may affect them. Prescribe rest and ice to reduce edema and inflammation. Tape or support the structures involved to allow mobility. As with all knee problems, correct all postural stresses where possible. Reassess the patient's activities, and alter habit patterns that may place stress on the structures.

Osgood-Schlatter Disease

Osgood-Schlatter disease is a condition that may start as a tendinitis of the patellar ligament at the tibial tubercle attachment, leading eventually to a separation of the epiphysis of the tubercle.[3,7,8,9,10] It may also occur as an injury separating the

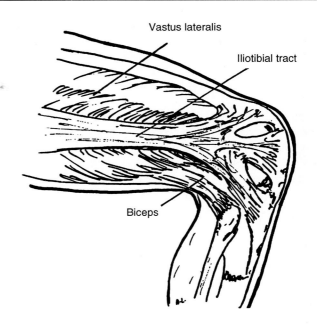

Vastus lateralis

Iliotibial tract

Biceps

Figure 6–44 Right knee, flexed, lateral view.

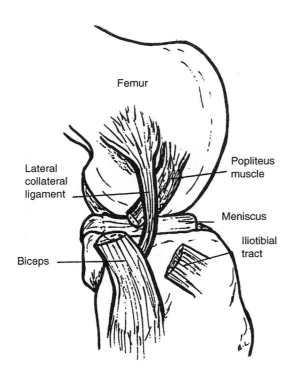

Figure 6–45 Right knee, lateral view.

epiphysis while running or jumping. It occurs most frequently in boys from 10 to 15 years of age.[3,7,8]

Palpation of the tibia tubercle usually reveals tenderness and an enlargement. Extension of the knee is usually painful; kneeling also produces pain.

X-ray examination will help differentiate among an avulsion fracture (the avulsed particle of the tubercle will appear a distance away toward the patella), the avulsed appearance of the normal apophysis, and Osgood-Schlatter disease. The last will show edema over the tuberosity; the infrapatellar fat pad will be blurred, the patellar ligament may be thickened, and the tubercle may be fragmented.[11]

Only in the extreme case, where complete tearing has occurred, is surgery called for. With rest and proper therapy, the symptoms usually disappear with closing of the epiphysis by age 20. Symptoms may continue on in the adult, however, if the patient continues with the same activities.

Ideally, patient compliance, rest, ice, refraining from activities that produce the symptoms, and time are all that is necessary to resolve the problem. Patient control is many times the biggest problem. Young boys may promise not to participate in activities, but one does not have to be in practice very long to realize that compliance is the exception rather than the rule. Peer pressure and short attention span may both be blamed.

The milder case, where pain is minimal without activity and patient compliance can be expected, requires less attention.

The author has had good success by applying elastic tape from the tibia to the midfemur, restricting flexion beyond that needed to walk. Even the patient who intends to refrain from activity will many times participate as a result of peer pressure. Taping sometimes acts as a reminder, and in some cases a badge, that there is really something wrong.

In cases where compliance is not expected, there are many supports and braces manufactured to prevent strain to the ligamental attachment.

Larsen-Johansson Disease

Osteochondritis of the patella at its tendon attachments occurs most often at the attachment of the patellar ligament on the inferior pole. The etiology is similar to that of Osgood-Schlatter disease, and the treatment is the same.

BURSITIS

Bursae around the knee are numerous (11 to 18 or more; Figures 6–46 and 6–47). Three bursae communicate with the joint; swelling and pain should call for further investigation into possible internal joint problems:

1. *suprapatellar bursa*: under the quadriceps tendon
2. *popliteus bursa:* between the popliteus tendon and the lateral condyle of the femur
3. *medial gastrocnemius bursa:* between the tendon and the capsule

Enlargement of the medial gastrocnemius bursa (Baker's cyst) is often associated with a torn meniscus. When present, full flexion of the knee is difficult and gives a feeling of fullness in the popliteal space. Extension produces tension in the space.

Bursitis may be caused by infections, but repeated falls and irritation are the most common causes. The patellar bursa lies in front of the lower half of the patella and the upper half of the patellar ligament. It may become inflamed from prolonged kneeling (housemaid's knee). It is easily palpated, and testing of the quadriceps will produce pain if it is inflamed. The pes anserinus bursa lies between the tibia and the tendons of the sartorius, gracilis, and semitendinosus muscles. It is easily palpated and produces pain upon testing of the muscles. The bursa under the medial collateral ligament may produce pain upon testing of the sartorius and gracilis but not necessarily upon testing of the semitendinosus. It may produce pain on valgus stressing of the slightly flexed knee. Careful palpation along the course of the medial ligament will reveal tenderness and edema.

Bursitis not of infectious origin will usually subside with rest, ice, and corrections of activities or stresses felt to be the cause. Ultrasound and other modalities to reduce pain and

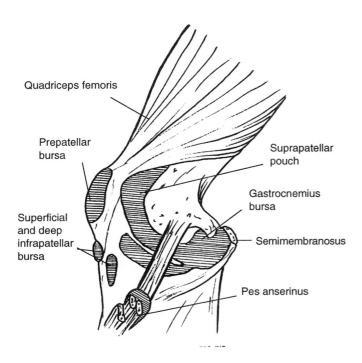

Quadriceps femoris

Prepatellar bursa

Superficial and deep infrapatellar bursa

Suprapatellar pouch

Gastrocnemius bursa

Semimembranosus

Pes anserinus

Figure 6–46 Right knee, medial view showing bursae.

edema are used in the treatment of bursitis. If, after reduction, the bursitis recurs, especially in bursae that communicate with the joint, investigation of the internal joint structure and the use of anti-inflammatory medications should be considered.

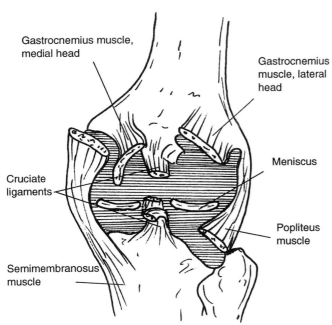

Gastrocnemius muscle, medial head

Gastrocnemius muscle, lateral head

Cruciate ligaments

Meniscus

Popliteus muscle

Semimembranosus muscle

Figure 6–47 Right knee, posterior view showing bursae.

CHONDROMALACIA PATELLA

Chondromalacia patella is defined as softening and degeneration of the articular surfaces of the patella, but the term is used to encompass the trochlear groove of the femur as well.

Symptoms include pain behind the patella, especially after sitting, and pain on climbing stairs or walking downstairs. Edema may be associated with the disease, and if present it is difficult to differentiate from a suprapatellar bursitis. There will be pain on testing of the QF and pain with pressure on the patella with the leg extended and the patient contracting the QF.

Cailliet[4] reports that studies done on normal knees have revealed a large number of asymptomatic chondromalacia cartilages. He further reports that other studies have found abnormal cartilages with increasing frequency as age increased, which indicates that changes begin usually at 20 years of age and are found in nearly everyone by age 35.

If the pain is caused by inflammation or degeneration on the patellar surface alone, with no other surfaces affected, pain would occur with pressure on the patella. Pain would occur in all degrees of flexion or extension. Careful palpation will help differentiate whether it is the patella alone, the trochlear groove, or both.

Plica

Kuland[6] states that in the embryo a septum separates the suprapatellar pouch from the major part of the knee joint. The septum usually disappears. Twenty percent of the time, however, it persists as a fibrous band (plica). It begins on the undersurface of the QF tendon just above the patella, extending transversely to insert on the medial wall of the knee joint.

Most are soft, pliable, and asymptomatic. When thickened, the plica is suspected as the cause of chondromalacia, is caused by the chondromalacia, or is associated with the disease as a result of other causes.

Etiology

The cause of chondromalacia is considered idiopathic by many investigators. Some associate it with patella instability and dislocation in a small percentage of patients. Cailliet[4] reports that trauma is implicated, but the exact cause remains unknown. Still others report findings and treatment programs but never discuss the cause.

Degenerative changes may result from the following:

- trauma (symptoms may have subsided, but imbalances caused by the injury or misuse during recovery have not been corrected)
- repetitive microtrauma with its associated inflammation (possibly from trauma)
- any postural distortion that produces abnormal movement of the patella in the trochlear groove

With a careful history and a thorough examination of the knee and the body as a whole, a correct diagnosis and the probable cause may be found.

Differentiation

Flex the knee to 100° and test the QF. In the same position, apply pressure to the patella. By flexing the knee to 110°, pressure is exerted on the undersurface of the patella and the inferior surface of the femoral condyle.

If pain is elicited by both testing the QF and applying pressure at 110°, it is reasonable to assume that chondromalacia patella exists. This would require investigation of the articular surface of the femoral condyle. If pain does not occur with pressure on the patella at 110° but does occur with the QF test, the chances are that the problem is in the trochlear groove and not the patella.

Bring the knee to 100° of flexion (this releases some muscle tension), and carefully palpate the entire trochlear groove for edema and pain (Figures 6–48 and 6–49).

Bring the knee to 40° and palpate the medial border of the patella, the medial rim of the trochlear groove, and the space between for an enlarged plica.

Whether findings indicate chondromalacia of the patella, chondromalacia of the trochlear groove, or inflammation of the plica, degeneration has taken place. Diagnosis is made on the basis of the symptoms associated with whatever degree of degeneration is present, not on the basis of degeneration alone. Besides the studies referred to earlier, Brashear and Raney[9] report that 50% of cadavers with supposedly normal knees show chondromalacia degeneration.

Treatment

The most severe cases may require surgery if conservative treatment fails, with removal of part or all of the cartilage. In some severe cases, the patella is removed.

Chiropractic approach to treatment should include the following:

- adjustment of all fixations that may affect function of the knee
- rest (this is one of the best treatments for any case with inflammation, yet sometimes it is the most difficult in terms of achieving patient compliance, especially in young patients)
- in the acute stage, ice to reduce edema
- support of the structures if necessary to assist in normal function
- low-wattage ultrasound over the trochlear groove (this has been useful in speeding recovery)
- at the earliest time possible, corrective exercises to resolve any postural faults that may be a causative factor

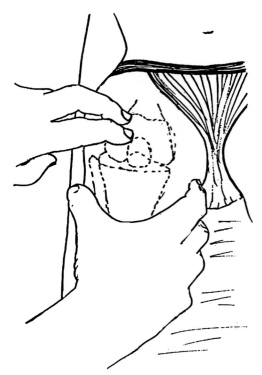

Figure 6–48 Palpation of the lateral trochlear wall.

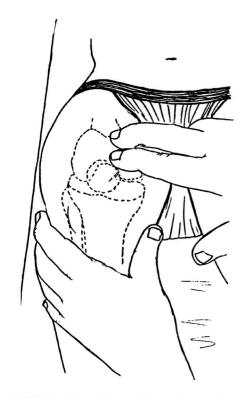

Figure 6–49 Palpation of the medial trochlear wall.

OSTEOCHONDRITIS DISSECANS

Osteochondritis dissecans is a separation of the cartilage with some subchondral bone from the articular surface of the femoral condyle. It occurs more often on the lateral side of the medial femoral condyle, and it affects children and young adults, mostly males.

Etiology

The disease may occur in children as an ossification anomaly (juvenile osteochondritis). It may also result from trauma, most cases being associated with unusually prominent spines of the tibial condyle. Violent medial rotation of a tibia with a prominent spine is considered the primary cause.

Symptoms

If the fragment has not completely separated, there will be pain in the medial knee that will be difficult to pinpoint. Light exercise may cause few or no symptoms. Heavy activity may start the pain. Pain may subside within 2 to 4 hours with rest, but there is usually residual stiffness.

If the fragment has completely separated and becomes a loose body, it may locate itself between the articular surfaces of the femur and tibia. If so, the knee will flex but will lock up as extension is attempted. This condition is usually accompanied by excessive fluid in the joint.

Diagnosis

Any locking of the knee must be investigated to determine whether a loose body exists within the joint. The fragment and/or its crater may be seen on plain films with the proper views. Further investigation may be done with use of arthrography, arthoscopic examination, and computed tomography.

Treatment

If the fragment is not loose and the articular surface is intact, rest and time may allow it to heal. If the stresses that may affect the condition have been removed and symptoms persist after 4 to 6 months, surgery should be considered.

If the knee locks and a loose body is suspected, manipulation may cause movement of the fragment from between the articular surfaces. With the patient seated and the knee relaxed at 90°, traction the knee toward the floor for a few moments, expanding the joint to the limit of its ligaments (Figure 6–50). Rotate the tibia laterally, and extend the knee (Figures 6–51 and 6–52). If this fails, rotate the tibial medially and extend the knee. It may be necessary to repeat several times until the fragment moves out of impingement.

LIGAMENT DAMAGE TO THE KNEE

Ligament damage may be classified as follows:

- *Mild*—A few fibers are torn, or there is tissue damage at the periosteal attachment, yet the integrity of the joint is intact. Careful palpation may reveal an area of pain and/or edema. Pain is produced upon stress of the ligament.
- *Moderate*—A greater number of fibers have been torn, allowing excessive movement of the joint. Damage is usually accompanied by edema. Movement or movement attempts may be inhibited by pain, edema, and the resulting contraction of the muscles. In the acute trauma case where pain and edema are present, it must be presumed that some degree of instability exists.
- *Severe*—There is complete tearing, or enough fibers are torn to allow great instability.

In the initial examination of acute trauma cases other than complete tears, the diagnosis of sprains to the ligaments and the meniscus can often be made in error.

Mild Sprains

Treatment of mild sprains comprises rest, ice for local edema, adjustment of all fixations that may affect knee function, and support (see taping procedures, Figures 6–28

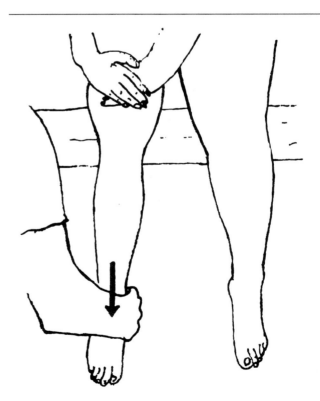

Figure 6–50 Treatment of loose body: apply traction toward the floor.

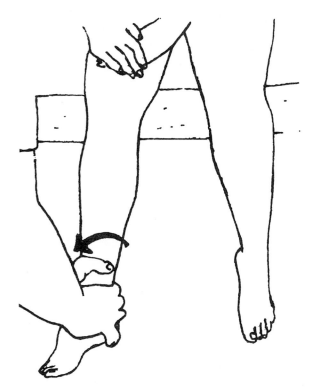

Figure 6–51 Treatment of loose body: rotate the tibia laterally.

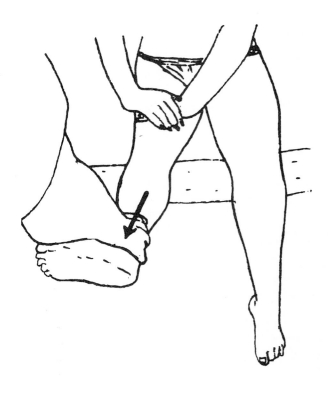

Figure 6–52 Treatment of loose body: extend the knee.

through 6–33 and Figures 6–35 through 6–37). Treatment should also be directed to other tissue damage that allowed the ligament damage to occur (ie, muscles, tendons, and fasciae). Rehabilitation exercises should be instituted to restore normal function and balance to the area.

Moderate Sprains

In the acute phase, moderate sprains must be assumed to be more severe than the examination reveals. Treatment involves rest, evaluation, and ice packs to reduce edema and pain. The edema should be reduced sufficiently to allow reevaluation of the extent of ligament damage within 72 hours.

Once it is ascertained that severe ligament damage is not present and that only minimal hypermobility is present, evaluation for meniscus tearing is also possible. When the edema is reduced, taping may be used for support, allowing mild exercises to be introduced (see taping procedures, Figures 6–28 through 6–33 and Figures 6–35 through 6–37).

Once the patient is able to bear weight with taping support (and, if necessary, a brace), ambulation may be gradually introduced, starting with crutches until the patient is stable. Rehabilitation exercises should always continue until function and strength are equal to those of the opposite limb. As long as any excessive joint play exists, exercises should be continued.

Severe Sprains

In the event that the anterior drawer sign is positive and hemarthrosis is present, the patient should be referred to an orthopedic surgeon for arthoscopic examination and, if necessary, surgery.

When complete tearing occurs, surgery is necessary to stabilize the knee. Where severe damage has occurred yet sufficient fibers exist, conservative care would include immobilization, elevation and ice, a full brace preventing movement, introduction of isometric exercises at the earliest time possible, exercises for the hip muscles and foot muscles to maintain strength and to aid in circulation, and exercises of the intact knee to take advantage of the cross-over effect. As the edema subsides and conditions allow, remove the brace three or four times per day, and introduce passive range of motion with progress to gentle active movement by the patient.

As progress allows, ambulation may be introduced at first with the aid of crutches, taping, and a brace. The use of support is necessary until sufficient stabilization has been achieved to return to normal activities. Even with the best results, a support during activities that would place undue stress on the knee is necessary.

It has been the author's experience that in the moderately severe sprain the procedures listed above have proven successful with a compliant patient. Although total strength of the ligament may not be achieved, overdevelopment of the musculature that secures the joint provides additional stability.

The severe sprain patient may never achieve full stability without surgical intervention and should have the options explained thoroughly. Patients may accept a change in their lifestyle and activities as well as the instability (with occasional "popping out") rather than undergo surgery. That is their privilege, and if, being fully informed of the possibilities, they wish to continue conservatively, they should be helped to the best of our ability.

It has also been the author's experience that the noncompliant patient, who reaches the stage of recovery where pain is no longer a factor and sufficient strength has returned to allow moderate activity, will usually discontinue the exercise program. This of course leaves the patient with a degree of instability and susceptible to reinjury. One of the most difficult tasks of the practitioner is to control patient behaviors until the maximum results are achieved.

MENISCUS TEARS

The medial meniscus is less mobile than the lateral meniscus because of its attachment on the periphery and the location of the tibial attachments anteriorly and posteriorly (Figures 6–53 and 6–54). The lateral meniscus is attached more centrally on the tibia without the peripheral attachments; thus it is more mobile.

Most tears occur when violent internal or external rotation of the femur occurs with the tibia fixed by weight bearing and the knee flexed. Both menisci move anteriorly during extension and posteriorly in flexion. In extreme flexion, the medial meniscus becomes compressed by the tibia and femur. During internal rotation of the femur with the tibia fixed, the posterior horn of the medial meniscus is displaced toward the center of the joint. If extension occurs suddenly, the posterior horn may become trapped, producing traction on the meniscus and possibly causing a longitudinal tear.

If external rotation and sudden extension occur, a transverse or oblique tear of the medial meniscus may be produced. If the tibia is fixed, the knee flexed, and valgus stress introduced, tearing of the peripheral attachment of the medial meniscus may occur. Also, possible tearing of fibers of the capsule and/or deep fibers of the medial collateral ligament may occur.

During flexion, the lateral meniscus is pulled posteriorly by the popliteus origin fibers, which also pull the posterior capsule out from impingement. Tears may occur in both the lateral and the medial menisci at several locations with the knee in various degrees of flexion when violent rotation takes place. Usually the greater the flexion at the time of injury, the more posterior the tear of the meniscus.

A torn meniscus must be suspected in any ligament injury. If it is not possible to investigate in the acute phase, the area should be investigated thoroughly as soon as possible.

The meniscus tissue is mostly avascular and will not heal. Only the vascular portion around the periphery will heal. The meniscus is lacking in sensory nerves. Therefore, pain associated with tearing is from other injured tissues and/or pressure from edema rather than from the meniscus itself.

Symptoms

Some tears are asymptomatic, as evidenced by the finding of old tears during surgery. Nevertheless, an injury sufficient to cause tearing must have had some symptoms at the time. Pain usually accompanies the injury, with the patient reporting that "something tore in the knee."

Swelling is caused by tearing of tissues other than the meniscus, making it necessary to investigate further. "Giving

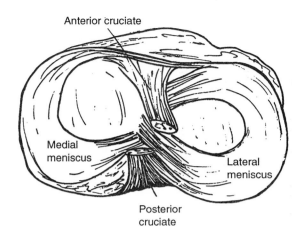

Figure 6–53 Right tibia, superior view.

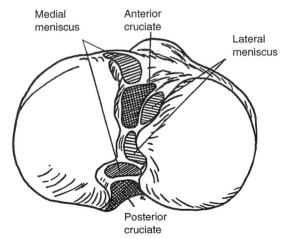

Figure 6–54 Structure of right tibia, superior view, showing menisci and ligament attachments.

way" during walking on an uneven surface or walking downstairs may occur (this is usually associated with a posterior tear). Locking seldom results from the initial injury. Locking may occur later with subsequent injuries that extend the tear farther forward or that tear away the particle, which then moves into the anterior joint.

Atrophy of the vastus medialis muscle is always mentioned as a sign soon after a meniscus injury. Of course, if the VMO was weak before the injury, it may have been partially responsible for the lack of stability. If not, it surely would become damaged during the injury, and this would become noticeable within a few days.

Treatment

Treatment includes rest, elevation and ice for effusion, and adjustment of all fixations that may affect knee function. If it is determined that a peripheral tear has occurred, the chance of full recovery is good because of the blood supply around the periphery.

One theory is that an injury may only "buckle" or crumple up the meniscus. If so, proper palpation and manipulation of the bony segments will replace the meniscus to its normal position and allow healing to occur.

After the effusion is reduced, careful palpation of the medial joint structure may reveal a small nodule (this will be extremely sensitive). If so, capsular fiber or collateral ligament tearing has allowed meniscus entrapment. The meniscus may be manipulated back into place to allow healing. With the patient in the supine position, sit on a stool approximately the same height as the table, facing footward. With the outside hand, grasp the ankle from underneath (Figure 6–55). Place the knee firmly against the operator's ilium (this prevents any pressure on the joint). With the fingers around and behind the knee, contact the nodule with a pisiform contact. The protrusion may be anterior or posterior of the midline of the meniscus.

The thrust is toward the center of the knee joint (see below); therefore, rotate the leg until the thrust is toward both the center of the joint and the operator's ilium. Traction the ankle laterally only as far as necessary to open the medial joint. This can be determined during palpation in preparation for the contact.

The thrust is given toward the center of the knee by the operator placing the elbow at 90° to the ilium. With a correct contact and the knee placed against the ilium, the thrust itself can do no harm to the knee structure. Therefore, the thrust may be sharp as the joint is opened up by traction on the ankle laterally.

As a follow-up, the author has found 3 minutes of ultrasound at approximately half power effective in promoting healing when coupled with 2 to 3 days of restricted flexion of the knee past 20°.

Although not as effective as the technique described above, the following alternative technique is useful in mild cases. With the patient supine, flex the hip and knee. Rotate the tibia (using the foot) medially (Figure 6–56A). This exposes the medial meniscus for each palpation. Apply pressure toward the center of the knee with a thumb contact on the suspected tissue while rotating the tibia laterally and extending the knee (Figure 6–56B).

If the tear is suspected to be internal, involving tissue that is avascular, conservative care may return the knee to normal function. There is a good possibility, however, that subsequent, relatively minor injuries will further tear the meniscus, making surgery necessary. Arthoscopic examination may provide not only an exact diagnosis but also the opportunity for surgical repair of the joint structures.

If the patient is informed of the options available and elects to avoid surgery, treatment should be continued with exercises, especially for the VMO, as soon as the pain and effusion have subsided. All postural stresses should be eliminated.

POSTSURGICAL PATIENTS

If the history and subsequent examination reveal a previous knee surgery, careful analysis of the knee and its present ability to function normally should be done.

A common finding is a history of surgery for a medial meniscus repair that was sufficiently successful to allow all symptoms to subside and a return to normal movement. Months or years later, however, the symptoms may appear without apparent reason or with minimal strain. One must keep in mind that surgery only repairs the obvious damage. It does nothing for the peripheral damage and/or the precipitating factors that had to occur to allow the meniscus tear in the first place.

It is not unusual for a patient to relate that he or she has had successful surgery, yet upon examination the knee is found to be in extreme hyperextension, and the VMO is half the bulk of the opposite leg (which may also be deficient). The surgeon

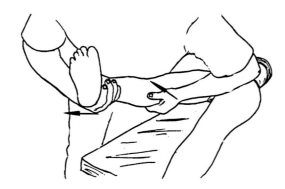

Figure 6–55 Maneuver for medial meniscus entrapment.

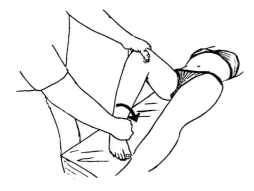
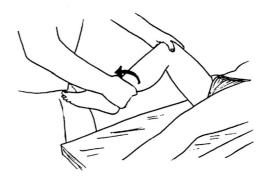

A   **B**

Figure 6–56 Alternative maneuver for medial meniscus entrapment. (**A**) Contacts. (**B**) Maneuver.

may not have prescribed the proper exercises for rehabilitation, or the patient failed to follow through as directed after the symptoms disappeared.

The primary complaint has to be addressed whether it requires surgery or not. Once the primary problem is on its way to being resolved, the patient must be made aware of what is necessary for recovery to the point where normal activities may be performed. The patient should also be fully informed of the consequences of not following through fully until complete stability is restored.

REFERENCES

1. Logan AL. *Diversified and Reflex Techniques Manual.* Los Angeles: Los Angeles Chiropractic College; 1974–1978.
2. Shafer RC. The knee involvement in foot pronation. In: Anderson JG, ed. *Clinical Biomechanics.* 2nd ed. Baltimore: Williams & Wilkins; 1987.
3. Greenwalt MH. *The Foot, Gait and Chiropractic.* Research Bulletin No. 699. Roanoke: Foot Levelers, Inc.; 1990.
4. Cailliet R. *Knee Pain and Disability.* Philadelphia: Davis; 1980.
5. Hoppenfeld S. *Physical Examination of the Spine and Extremities.* New York: Appleton-Century-Crofts; 1976.
6. Kuland DN. *The Injured Athlete.* Philadelphia: Lippincott; 1988.
7. Souza T. Evaluating lateral knee pain. *Chirop Sports Med.* 1989;3.
8. Kapandji IA. *The Physiology of the Joints.* New York: Churchill Livingstone; 1977.
9. Brashear HR, Raney RB. *Handbook of Orthopaedic Surgery.* St Louis: Mosby; 1986.
10. Turek S. *Orthopaedics: Principles and Their Applications.* Philadelphia: Lippincott; 1967.
11. Yochum T. *Essentials of Skeletal Radiology.* Vols. 1,2. Baltimore: Williams & Wilkins; 1986.

Chapter 7

Exercises and Stretches

Exercise is important in prevention of problems, recovery from trauma, and rehabilitation to preinjury status and beyond.

Trauma or symptoms make it necessary for patients to present themselves for treatment, with success being measured by the cessation of symptoms and the return to normal. Normal, of course, may not be what is correct.

If examination reveals abnormal posture or poor habit patterns, the practitioner should make sure that the patient is fully informed of the problem and provide a treatment program.

Not only must the patient with a chronic postural fault be introduced to corrective exercises, but the practitioner must look further into the habit patterns of activities during work or recreation and advise the patient in altering the activity. Habit patterns are often difficult to overcome. As an example, patients with a chronic laterally rotated femur develop a gait with the foot turned out. If the cause is corrected and medial rotator exercises seem to be effective, then the habit pattern should be altered. One method used by the author is to have the patient walk down the hall in the office for 40 to 50 steps, following these instructions:

1. Carefully place the heel on the floor (this requires the patient to look down at the feet during the entire exercise).
2. Deliberately place the forefoot in front without allowing rotation to occur.
3. *Slowly* and *deliberately* place the weight on the heel and then on the forefoot.
4. Follow with the opposite foot.

Each stride must be observed by the patient, otherwise he or she will revert to old habits. This alteration technique should be performed at least twice per day for 3 to 4 days until the habit pattern is broken.

Patients who have experienced trauma should be given exercises to restore muscle function as soon as practical. In the severe stage, when edema and pain are present, exercises may be harmful. As soon as the edema is reduced, however, exercises may be introduced with caution.

If ligament damage has occurred that does not require surgery, taping to reinforce the joint structure is a necessity before introducing an exercise. Always start with mild exercises, increasing as symptoms will allow, for the muscles that produce the movement that reduces the strain on the injured ligament structure. As an example, for medial collateral ligament injury, once taping to reinforce the joint structure and the oblique fibers of the vastus medialis (VMO) has been placed and the edema is gone, exercises may begin. With ligament laxity being a possibility after healing has taken place, many times overdevelopment of the musculature may be necessary to stabilize the knee.

Two types of exercise may be used: isometric, in which there is no joint movement, only contraction of the musculature; and isotonic, in which there is active movement against resistance.

Isotonic exercise may be performed with weights or with resistant material such as stretchable tubing.

Getting patients to perform exercises at home is, at best, difficult. Getting a patient to do the *correct* exercises at home is even more difficult. It is easy and simple to hand out a set of standard exercises for a patient to perform, but such a practice is fraught with problems. For one, unless designed specifically for the problem the particular patient is experiencing, some of the exercises may be harmful. Also, without actually going through the exercises while supervised by the practitioner, the patient usually has difficulty in figuring out exactly how to perform them. Further, if the patient performs the exercise incorrectly or does the wrong exercise, the condition may deteriorate, with the patient getting discouraged and not returning. If and when the patient does return, it is still necessary to review the exercises. Therefore, it is more efficient to rehearse the patient to start with.

It has been the author's experience that, to ensure that exercises are performed correctly, the following should be done:

1. Give a careful description in lay terms of exactly what the problem is.
2. Test the muscle, and demonstrate to the patient how weak it is and why exercise is necessary.
3. Demonstrate the exercise.
4. Have the patient perform the exercise, making sure that cheating (recruitment of other muscles) does not occur.
5. Provide, where possible, a drawing of the exercise to be used as a reminder.
6. Make exercise tubing available if it is to be used. Do not rely on the patient's purchasing this somewhere else.
7. If a spouse is available, recruit him or her to assist in reminding the patient to do the exercises and to observe whether they are being done correctly.
8. Explain exactly how many repetitions at each session and how many sessions per day are expected.
9. On the following visit, review the results and have the patient repeat the exercise to ensure that it is being performed correctly.

Where possible, performance of the exercise in the office with a return to the office in 2 to 3 days just to perform the exercise will ensure that exercises are being performed and, more important, that they are being performed correctly.

Stretchable tubing has been used by the author for many years. There are several brands of tubing currently on the market. Stretchable tubing allows a patient to perform exercises at home, at work, or while traveling.

A length of about 5 ft will allow most exercises to be performed. Tie a knot in each end of the tubing, and the exercises may begin. If a bicycle inner tube is used, cut out the stem.

Why use tubing? Why not just send the patient to a gym or fitness center for exercises? First, some patients cannot afford to join. Second, some of the acute patients could not go. Third, most would not go more than once per day, and most would

perform the exercises only three or four times per week. Finally, with tubing and proper instructions provided, patients may do the exercises as many times per day as needed.

Active participation of the patient in the treatment process is essential. Patient attitude all too often is one of placing all the responsibility on the practitioner. After the initial diagnosis and treatment during the acute stage, patient participation is a must if complete rehabilitation is to be accomplished.

All the exercises described and illustrated in this chapter have been used with success for many years by the author.

LORDOTIC LUMBAR SYNDROME

The lordotic lumbar syndrome (Figure 7–1) is one of the most common postural distortions with knee strain found in practice. Knee pain is only one of the many symptoms associated with it. The anterior rotation of the pelvis and increased lordosis of the lumbar spine must be reduced before exercises for the lateral rotators of the hip will be effective. As long as these exist, the Q angle will remain increased as a result of the medial rotation of the femur (Figure 7–2).

Note: Below and elsewhere in this chapter, the exercises call for the use of weight, a certain number of repetitions per session, and a certain number of sessions per day. The practitioner must prescribe these individually, according to each patient's injury and each injury's severity.

The patient with lordotic lumbar syndrome should be instructed in the following exercise:

1. Lie on the floor, a couch, or a bed.
2. Place the prescribed amount of weight on the abdomen below the umbilicus.
3. Bend one knee as shown in Figure 7–3, and using that leg only raise the buttocks off the surface while rotating the pelvis (move the pubic bone toward the chin). Hold for 5 to 6 seconds, then return to the table slowly.
4. Repeat six to eight times, then repeat on the opposite side.
5. Compare one side with the other, and if one takes more effort repeat the exercise on that side six to eight more times.
6. The above constitutes one session. You should perform at least the prescribed number of sessions per day.

The weight on the abdomen is an important part of the exercise. When asked to do the exercise without weight, the patient usually will *increase* the lumbar curve. Patients who are obese or who cannot raise the buttocks off the table many times may be able to do so if the operator applies hand pressure of 5 to 10 pounds on the abdomen. The weight seems to trigger a reflex to rotate the pelvis posteriorly, allowing raising to occur.

Some general exercises for the lower back include raising the buttocks using both legs. If done, this exercise *increases* the lordosis of the lumbar spine.

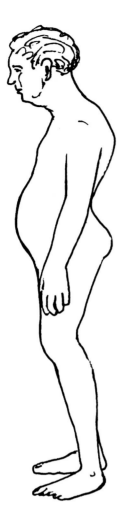

Figure 7–1 Lordotic lumbar syndrome.

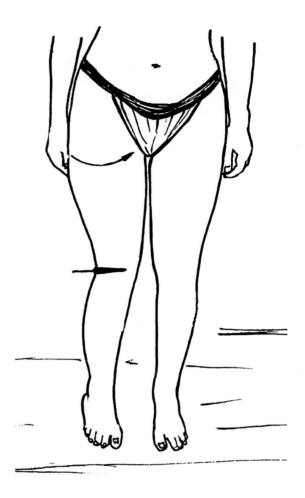

Figure 7–2 Valgus knee and medially rotated femur (increased Q angle).

Female patients who have had children must be screened for abdominal muscles that not only may be weak but may have ceased functioning during the later stages of pregnancy. Abdominal muscle function and tone must be reestablished. To accomplish this, have the patient perform a bilateral straight leg raise (Figure 7–4). Observe the pelvis at the start of the effort. As the hip flexors contract, the abdominal muscles should contract, securing the pelvis to provide a fulcrum for the function. If the abdominals are weak, the pelvis will rotate anteriorly before the legs leave the table. To prove the necessity of doing the exercises, place your hand on the lower abdominal area and help function by stabilizing the pelvis (Figure 7–5). The legs will raise more easily.

In women who have had children, reestablishing the habit pattern of abdominal muscle function takes effort and patience on the operator's part. With the patient supine, place one hand underneath the patient on the sacrum. With the other hand contact the lower abdomen, and physically rotate the pelvis

posteriorly several times to show the patient what is expected. Then have the patient start helping in the movement, and then have her do it herself: Stop, remove the hands, and ask the patient to perform the same function. Most of the time she cannot; everything except the pelvis may move. Assistance should be provided again and the process repeated. The patient may think that she is performing the movement when in fact

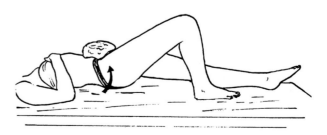

Figure 7–3 Lordosis exercise.

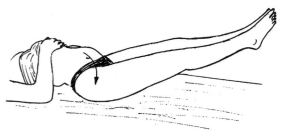

Figure 7–4 Bilateral straight leg raise with pelvic rotation.

the pelvis does not move. Have the patient place her hand on the pubic area so she may feel the lack of movement during the attempt.

Instruct the patient to attempt to rotate the pelvis at home 10 times per session for three sessions per day and to return in 2 days. Some patients may return and are able to rotate the pelvis. Most require at least one more session in the office with assistance before the habit pattern in reestablished.

Having the patient compare one side with the other for the amount of effort to perform is a simple way of achieving balance of the muscles.

Sit-ups are also useful for the patient with lordotic lumbar syndrome. Instruct the patient as follows:

1. Lie on the floor with the legs on a chair. Make sure that the hip is flexed to 90°.

2. With arms outstretched, try to rise up and touch an imaginary point to your extreme right (Figure 7–6A); this is position 1 of the exercise. Hold, then slowly return to the floor. Repeat progressively across to your extreme left (Figure 7–6B); this is position 6 of the exercise. Rest, then repeat back from position 6 to position 1.

3. After all 12 sit-ups have been performed, compare position 1 with position 6. If one takes more effort than the other, repeat that one an additional three to four times. Then compare position 2 with position 5, then position 3 with position 4, and repeat each one that takes more effort an additional three to four times.

4. The above constitutes one session. Perform the prescribed number of sessions per day.

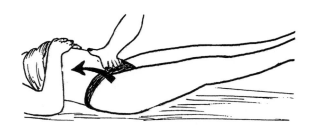

Figure 7–5 Bilateral straight leg raise with support.

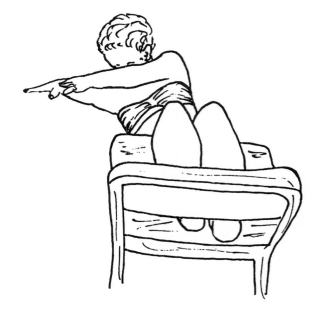

A

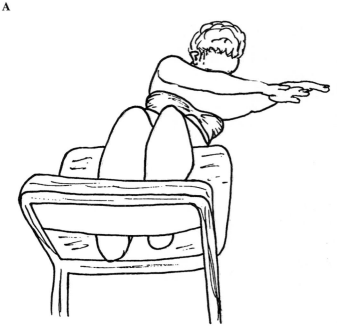

B

Figure 7–6 Sit-ups. **(A)** Position 1. **(B)** Position 6. The patient moves progressively across the body from position 1 to position 6 and back.

By having the hips flexed at 90°, most of the function of the psoas muscle is removed from participation (usually the psoas is hypertonic and/or shortened). Using 6 positions exercises all the abdominal muscles. The extreme outside positions exercise the transverse abdominus muscles.

GLUTEUS MAXIMUS MUSCLE

Exercise 1

Instruct the patient in the following exercise to strengthen the gluteus maximus:

1. On all fours, bend one knee and push the foot toward the ceiling (Figure 7–7). Do not move the pelvis. The thigh does not normally move more than 10° beyond neutral. If moved beyond 10°, the pelvis must rotate to allow it, which would defeat the purpose of the exercise. Start with 8 to 10 repetitions on each side, then compare. If one side takes more effort than the other, repeat on that side six to eight more times.
2. The above constitutes one session. You should perform the prescribed number of sessions per day.

As strength improves, ankle weights or a heavy boot may be added, and the number of repetitions may be increased.

Exercise 2

The next exercise uses tubing:

1. Standing next to the corner of a desk or table, place the front of the upper thigh of the weight-bearing leg against the desk for support. Flex the hip and knee on the side to be exercised.
2. Place the tubing around the foot, securing the ends on the desk with both hands (Figure 7–8).
3. Against the resistance, push the foot back, moving the knee no farther than 6 to 8 in past the other knee.
4. Repeat six to eight times, then change positions and repeat on the opposite side.
5. If one side requires greater effort to perform, repeat the exercise on that side four to five additional times.

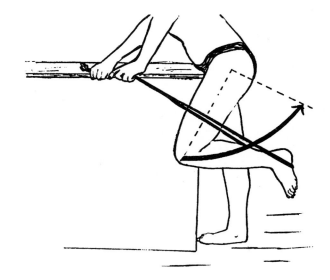

Figure 7–8 Standing gluteus maximus exercise.

Exercise 3

The following is a good exercise for patients with other injuries or problems that make it preferable to do exercises in non–weight bearing positions:

1. While lying on the floor, a couch, or a bed, either secure the tubing to an object or hold the ends.
2. Place the tubing around the foot with the hip and knee flexed (Figure 7–9).
3. Against the resistance, push the foot, bringing the knee toward the surface. Repeat six to eight times.
4. Repeat on the opposite side, and then compare. If one side requires greater effort than the other, repeat on that side an additional six to eight times.

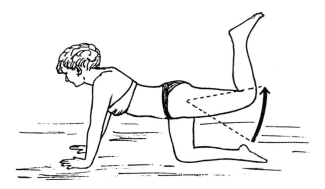

Figure 7–7 Gluteus maximus exercise.

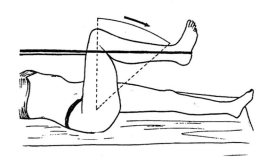

Figure 7–9 Supine gluteus maximus exercise.

LATERAL HIP ROTATOR MUSCLES

These exercises include the piriformis and gluteal muscles.

Exercise 1

1. Secure the tubing to the leg of a couch or other heavy furniture on the side to be exercised. You should exercise the prescribed side(s) (right, left, or both).
2. Sit slumped in a chair with the hip extended to approximately 30°. Do not sit up straight (Figure 7–10).
3. Against resistance, move the foot toward the opposite side (this rotates the thigh laterally).
4. Repeat 8 to 10 times.
5. Change positions and repeat on the opposite side if prescribed. Compare the amount of effort required; if one side requires more effort, repeat on that side an additional 6 to 8 times.

The piriformis muscle becomes an abductor of the hip when the hip is flexed to 90°. Therefore, it is mandatory that the exercise be performed with the hip extended to at least 30°.

Exercise 2

1. Sit up straight.
2. Secure the tubing around the lower thigh and/or knee with the other end secured to the opposite knee (Figure 7–11).

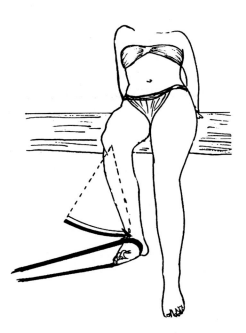

Figure 7–10 First piriformis exercise.

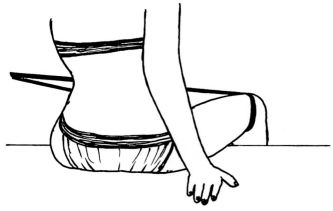

Figure 7–11 Second piriformis exercise.

3. Against resistance, move the knee to the side.
4. Repeat six to eight times.

QUADRICEPS FEMORIS AND OBLIQUE FIBERS OF THE VASTUS MEDIALIS

General exercises are excellent for the individual who does not have a deficiency, but if a demand is made for the quadriceps femoris (QF) to function and stretching or injury prevents the VMO from doing its part, the exercise will perpetuate the imbalance that exists. The functioning muscles will get stronger while the nonfunctioning VMO may even get weaker or stretch further, leading to further imbalance and the inevitable consequences. A careful analysis of the imbalance and guidance in the exercise program are necessary.

The following exercises cover most of the conditions encountered.

Exercise 1

1. If QF exercise is called for and the knee cannot be flexed (because of surgery or chondromalacia), place the intact limb across the ankle of the side to be exercised. Attempt to perform a straight leg raise, with the other limb providing the weight for resistance (Figure 7–12).
2. If the VMO is to be emphasized, rotate the leg laterally and attempt the straight leg raise. Once the VMO and other quadriceps muscles secure the knee, only attempt to elevate slightly. Further elevation only exercises the hip flexors.

Exercise 2

As the patient improves and some flexion is allowed, a pillow may be placed under the lower thigh, allowing slight flexion (Figure 7–13). The exercise is the same as exercise 1, ex-

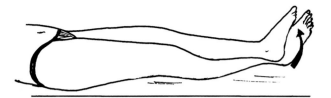

Figure 7–12 Isometric QF exercise.

cept that the use of the pillow allows the last few degrees of extension to be performed.

Exercise 3

If the patient is unable to sit or stand to perform exercises, the QF exercise with an emphasis on the VMO may be performed as follows:

1. Secure the tubing around the foot and cross it over the ankle.
2. With the hip and knee flexed and the knee allowed to move to the side, secure the ends of the tubing with your hand (Figure 7–14A).
3. Against resistance, extend the leg and move the knee to the opposite side at the same time in one smooth movement (Figure 7–14B).

To emphasize the vastus lateralis, start with the knee toward the opposite side, and move it to the side with extension.

Exercise 4

If the patient cannot exercise sitting or standing, all the QF muscles may be exercised on both limbs at once:

1. Flex the hips and knees.
2. Place the tubing under the feet.
3. Secure the tubing ends by hand.
4. Extend the knees, moving from a position with the knees to the left and in progressive positions to the right (Figure 7–15). This exercises all the QF muscles, not just the rectus femoris and vastus intermedialis.

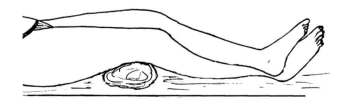

Figure 7–13 QF exercise with minimal flexion.

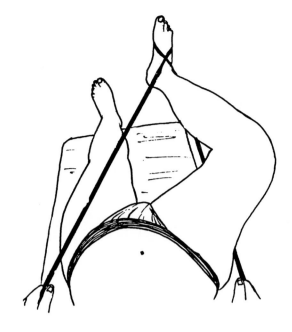

A

B

Figure 7–14 Supine VMO exercise. **(A)** Start. **(B)** Finish.

Exercise 5

The same exercise as exercise 3 may be performed if the patient is able to sit (Figure 7–16).

Exercise 6

Once the patient can bear weight, a simple exercise may be performed by standing on the limb to be exercised and holding onto a doorknob or other object to maintain balance. Obviously, all the body weight is used when the knee is flexed. In

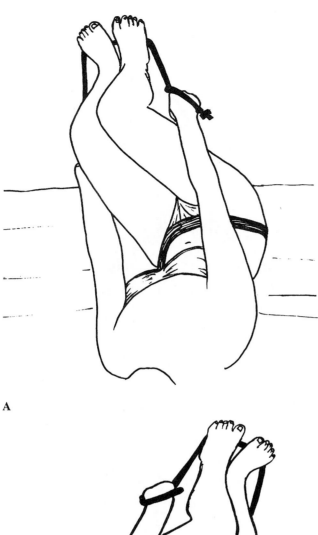

A

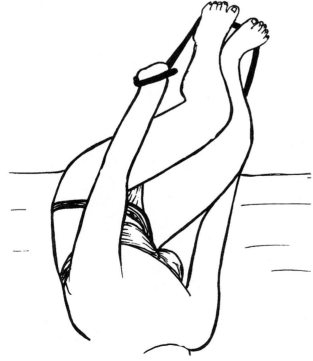

B

Figure 7–15 Supine QF exercise. (**A**) Start. (**B**) Finish.

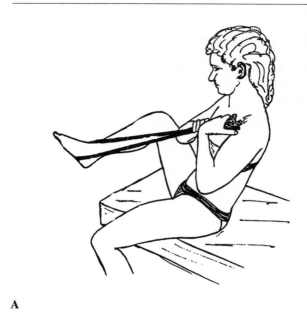

A

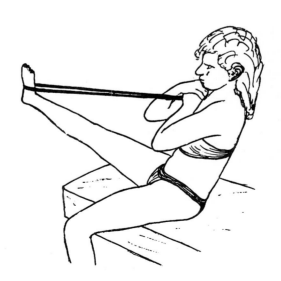

B

Figure 7–16 Sitting VMO exercise. (**A**) Start. (**B**) Finish.

the beginning and with elderly patients, leave the other foot on the floor, bearing weight sufficient to prevent falling or straining. As the patient improves, the supporting foot may be removed completely from the floor.

1. Stand on the prescribed foot, turning it inward slightly, and rotate the pelvis laterally as far as comfortable (Figure 7–17).
2. Bend the knee only to tolerance (in the beginning, only 10° to 15°). As strength is gained, increase the flexion, going farther and farther into a squat. (Most practitioners believe that the VMO is only utilized in the last 10° to 15° of extension. As discussed in Chapter 3, however, the use of the VMO throughout the entire range of motion has been proven clinically.)
3. After 8 to 10 knee bends, rotate the pelvis medially and repeat.

The VMO may be worked greater with the foot rotated laterally (Figure 7–18), but most injuries also include the popliteus muscle; therefore, the exercises should begin with medial rotation of the foot. Once the patient feels secure, exercise in both medial and lateral rotation.

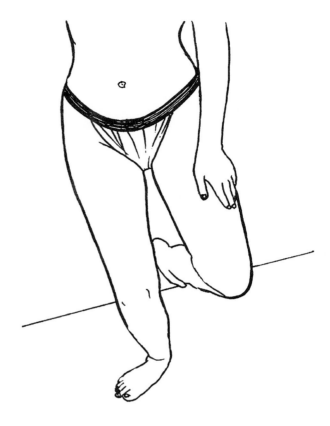

Figure 7–18 Knee bend exercise for the VMO with foot turned outward.

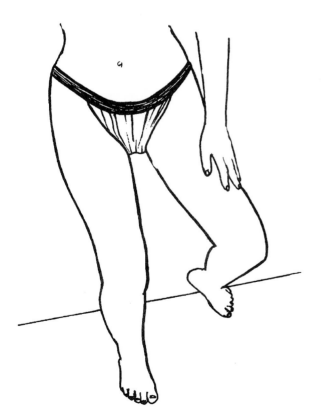

Figure 7–17 Knee bend exercise for the VMO with foot turned inward.

Exercise 7

One of the most common QF injuries occurs during skiing. A frequent factor that allows accidents to happen (other than recklessness) is fatigue and then overexertion of the muscles.

Typically, a skier has a desk job all summer and fall and then, when the snow falls, decides immediately to go skiing with no conditioning of the muscles. The same individual may arrive on the slopes early in the morning and not quit until late afternoon, doing activities that may overtax the muscles in the first hour.

Experienced skiers do not normally just go straight down the slope. Most of the strength in skiing is from the QF with the knees bent. When movement to the side is required, stress is placed on the vastus lateralis of one limb and the vastus medialis (and especially the VMO) of the other.

With the VMO weak to start with in some postural faults, fatigue sets in quickly and with further stress it gives out, allowing damage to the rest of the knee structure (Figure 7–19).

Exercises for the QF with straight extension, whether an apparatus is used or not, exercise all the QF. As stated earlier in this chapter, this often increases the disparity of the muscles.

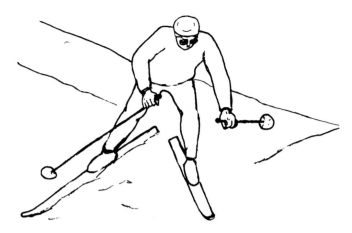

Figure 7–19 QF fatigue in skiing.

To prevent this from happening, the following exercise is useful in preparing the skier for the slopes; it is also useful for overall conditioning of any patient:

1. Stand on the tubing (stronger persons may require two or more tubes), squat, and secure the ends by hand.

2. Against the resistance, attempt to rise to standing at first with the knees to the left and progressively moving to the right (Figure 7–20).

3. This conditions all the QF muscles. If the exercise is more difficult to perform in one of the positions, the exercise should be repeated in that position until equal.

Exercise 8

For the patient who works out in the gym, the QF apparatus may be used. Rotating the thigh medially (Figure 7–21A) and then laterally (Figure 7–21B) while pushing the lever in the same direction, however, will emphasize the VMO and vastus lateralis, respectively.

Stretches

In the elderly patient, where bending, squatting, and other activities involving extreme knee flexion are no longer performed, it is not unusual to find a shortened QF. Elderly patients who have been treated with injections of cortisone for knee pain must be suspected of having this problem because it is a common reaction.

If the patient is unable to stand, the stretch may be performed lying down on a bed, couch, or table with the limb to be stretched off the side. Instruct the patient to grasp the ankle and pull the heel to the buttocks, allowing the knee to drop below the surface (Figure 7–22). This stretches all the QF muscles, including the rectus femoris, which crosses the hip joint.

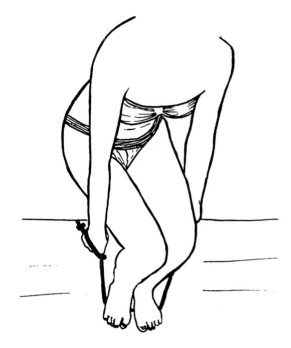

A

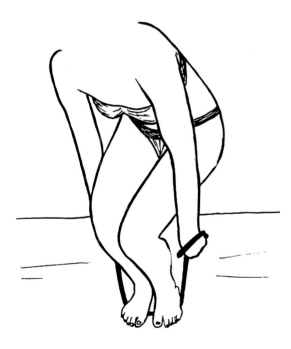

B

Figure 7–20 Exercise to strengthen all QF muscles for skiing. (**A**) Start. (**B**) Finish.

If the patient can stand, the stretch may be performed conveniently and thus more often, which will produce results more quickly (Figure 7–23). The patient may also use the opposite hand to apply the pressure.

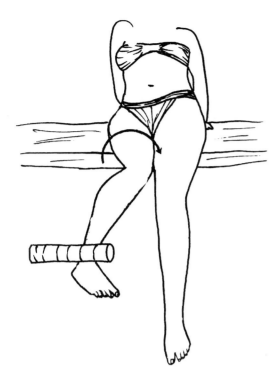

A

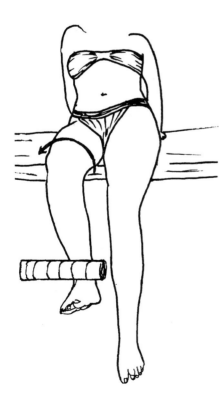

B

Figure 7–21 QF exercises on apparatus. (**A**) Thigh medially rotated to emphasize the VMO. (**B**) Thigh laterally rotated to emphasize the vastus lateralis.

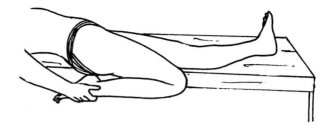

Figure 7–22 Supine QF stretch.

Another method, although not as effective, is to have the patient, with the leg extended, apply pressure distally on the patella using a thumb web contact, holding until a release is felt (Figure 7–24).

POPLITEUS MUSCLE

As indicated earlier in this text, a common error in testing the popliteus muscle is testing it with the knee at 90°. Patients with short medial hamstrings and patients with chronic popliteal weakness who have used the medial hamstrings to make up for this weakness may test normal at 90°, yet when the knee is moved farther into flexion a weakened popliteus will be displayed.

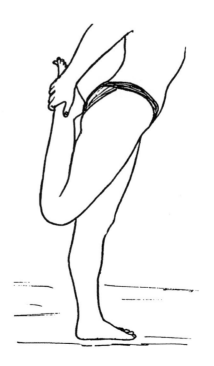

Figure 7–23 Standing QF stretch.

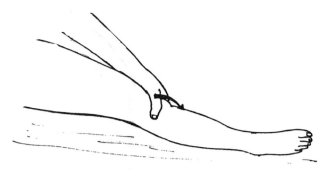

Figure 7–24 Alternative QF stretch.

Exercise 1

1. By sitting on a low stool, the knee is flexed beyond 90°, making the popliteus muscle perform without great benefit from the medial hamstrings.
2. Secure the tubing laterally and around the forefoot in lateral rotation (Figure 7–25A).
3. Against resistance and with the heel on the floor and the knee held still, rotate the foot medially. Do not invert the foot (Figure 7–25B).

Exercise 2

An isometric exercise may be performed by placing the opposite foot forward. With the forefoot against the opposite heel, the patient attempts medial rotation, making sure that the heel stays on the floor and the knee stays still (Figure 7–26).

For patients who work in an office, a variation of this exercise may be performed using the rung of a chair to anchor the heel with the opposite leg providing the resistance. If a secretary chair is used, the heel may be placed above the wheel mounting with the knee flexed sufficiently to perform the exercise.

HAMSTRING MUSCLES

Exercises

With the tubing secured in front, the patient hooks the heel over the tubing and flexes against the resistance (Figure 7–27). By laterally rotating the thigh (bringing the foot medial), the lateral hamstring is emphasized (Figure 7–28). To exercise the medial hamstrings, the patient rotates the thigh medially. For the bedridden patient, or if preferred, the exercise may be performed in the prone position (Figure 7–29).

Stretches

1. Stand with the prescribed foot placed on a chair and a hand placed on the knee, securing it in extension. Lean

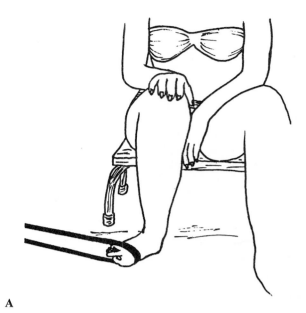

A

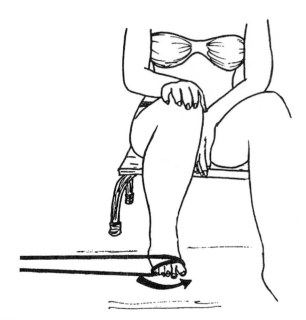

B

Figure 7–25 Popliteus muscle exercise. **(A)** Start. **(B)** Finish.

forward, with an emphasis on movement of the hip joint rather than the spine, until the hamstrings are tight (Figure 7–30). Avoid placing pressure great enough to cause pain.

2. Hold the position without any movement until relaxation is felt. Then move slightly farther into flexion,

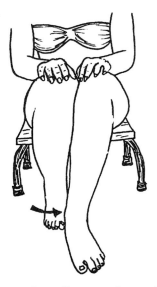

Figure 7–26 Isometric popliteus muscle exercise.

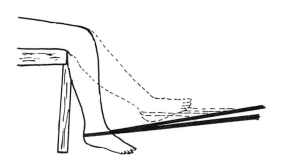

Figure 7–27 Hamstring muscle exercise.

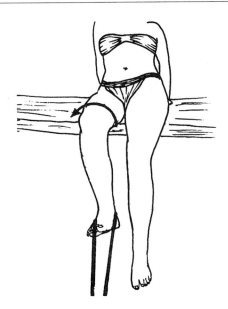

Figure 7–28 Exercise for the lateral hamstring.

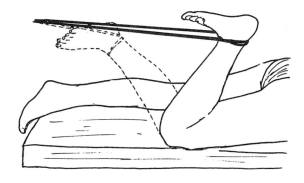

Figure 7–29 Prone hamstring exercise.

applying more stretch to the muscles. Again, hold still until relaxation is felt.

3. When stretched sufficiently, do not quit the position quickly. Gradually release the pressure.

For patients with back problems and the elderly, who may have difficulty standing on one leg, the following is probably a more efficient method. Instruct the patient to sit on the floor backed up against a wall. The patient places the heel on a stool and applies pressure to the knee to stretch the hamstrings (Figure 7–31). As hamstring length increases, a higher stool may be used.

TRICEPS SURAE MUSCLES

Seldom does the gastrocnemius muscle need exercising. Usually the dorsiflexors of the foot are the weak ones, and the

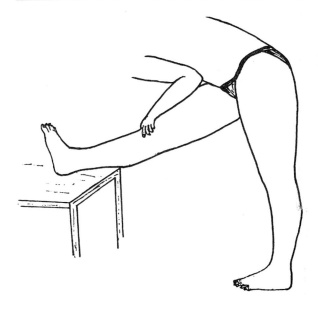

Figure 7–30 Standing hamstring muscle stretch.

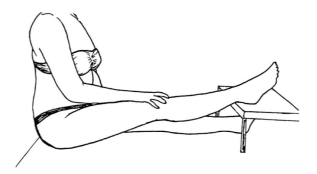

Figure 7–31 Sitting hamstring muscle stretch.

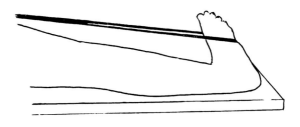

Figure 7–33 Sitting gastrocnemius stretch.

gastrocnemius is short or hypertonic. Occasionally it may test weak when the posterior tibialis muscle is weak or when pain exists from bursitis. To exercise the muscle, the patient simply stands and raises up on the toes.

One method used to stretch the gastrocnemius is to move the opposite foot forward into full stride. Using the weight of the body as it shifts back, the patient applies pressure and places the heel on the floor (Figure 7–32). This stretch has two components: pressure with the knee extended, and pressure with the knee flexed (to isolate the soleus muscle).

Another stretch is performed in the sitting position with the leg extended and uses a belt or tubing. With hand pressure, the patient pulls the foot into dorsiflexion to stretch the muscle (Figure 7–33).

The most effective method the author has found is to use a small slant board (13 × 3 in, rising from the floor to 5½ in; Figure 7–34). A patient with short gastrocnemius muscles cannot freestand on the board. The patient is forced into flex-

ing the hips and back to maintain balance. When the board is placed in a convenient location, the patient may stand on it several times per day, for example while watching television. In the beginning, 1 to 2 minutes is long enough. The length of time is gradually extended as the muscle lengthens. The process may take 3 to 4 weeks with some patients.

SARTORIUS AND GRACILIS MUSCLES

Instruct the patient as follows:

1. Secure the tubing around the leg of a piece of heavy furniture, in front of and approximately 40° lateral to you. Hook the heel into the loop, and against the re-

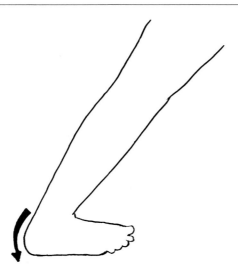

Figure 7–32 Standing gastrocnemius stretch.

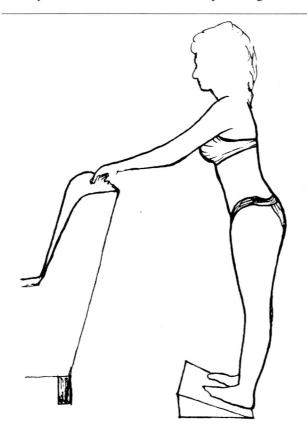

Figure 7–34 Slant board stretch for gastrocnemius muscle.

sistance attempt to move the ankle over the opposite knee (Figure 7–35).

2. Ankle weights may be used in the standing position. Stand with the knees wide apart with the body weight on the opposite foot. Bring the weighted ankle up and over the opposite knee (Figure 7–36). This exercise is not as effective as the preceding one.

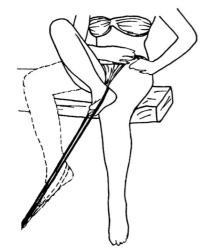

Figure 7–35 Sitting exercise for sartorius and gracilis.

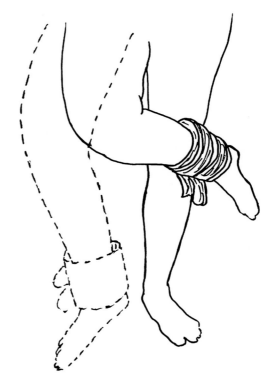

Figure 7–36 Standing exercise for sartorius and gracilis.

This chapter presents several case histories of patients with knee complaints and their progress. The author does not intend to give the impression that every patient treated responds to therapy. Some patients are beyond conservative care. Some patients are noncompliant and end up needing surgery that perhaps could have been prevented.

With a thorough examination, the correct diagnosis, and a cooperative patient, conservative care will usually remedy the immediate problem. Conservative care may also prevent problems in the future, some seemingly unrelated to the knee.

CASE 1

A 41-year-old man presented with the primary complaint of pain in the right knee on rising to stand and walking downstairs; he reported that it felt as though the knee would give way because of pain while he was walking. Pain during the night required him to get up and move around. Sometimes the pain was relieved sufficiently with analgesics to allow return to sleep.

History revealed that he had slipped on the left foot and fallen, catching all his body weight on the bent right leg. Upon examination by his family physician, the patient was radiographed and prescribed medication for pain.

Examination

All orthopedic tests were negative. The sartorius muscle tested weak with pain; it was not improved with manual support. Edema was detected on palpation under the pes anserinus muscle attachments. A match head nodule was palpated anterior to the medial collateral ligament.

Diagnosis

A minor tear of the periphery of the medial meniscus and fibers of the capsule with entrapment of the meniscus was diagnosed. Possible trauma to the pes anserinus or bursitis from $4\frac{1}{2}$ months of misuse of the knee was suspected.

Treatment

Adjustments were made of the lower back, pelvis, ankle, and foot as well as of the protruded meniscus. Low-wattage ultrasound was applied for 3 minutes. Ice therapy was applied to the pes anserinus. The knee was taped, not so much for support as to secure the knee to constrain movement past 20° of flexion.

Progress

Reevaluation on day 3 revealed greatly reduced pain both at the pes anserinus and in the joint itself. On day 14 after the onset of treatment, the patient was released free of pain. There were no painful areas on palpation, and all muscles tested normal.

CASE 2

A 52-year-old male attorney presented with the primary complaint of lower back pain for 25 years that never went away for more than 3 or 4 days no matter who treated him. He had received treatment from both medical doctors and chiropractors over the years. A secondary complaint was mild pain in the right knee from an old football injury at 18 years of age.

History revealed that he had been diagnosed with and treated for chondromalacia.

Examination

Pressure on the patella produced minimal pain in the extended knee. Tests of the quadriceps femoris (QF) elicited shakiness at most positions; pain was noted at 120° of flexion. With manual support of the patella medially the pain was reduced by 20% to 30%. The oblique fibers of the vastus medialis (VMO) were lacking in bulk visibly and on palpation.

Diagnosis

The diagnosis was chondromalacia, mild in the upper trochlear groove and severe along the medial border of the lateral femoral articular surface. Lateral tracking of the patella also was diagnosed, as was lower back pain (partly caused by or aggravated by the malfunctioning knee).

Treatment

All fixations relating to the condition were adjusted. Exercises were prescribed for a stretched quadratus lumborum muscle on the right (probably caused by the physiologic short right leg). Tape support and exercises for the VMO also were applied.

Progress

The tape was removed after 8 days; it was no longer necessary as long as the patient was careful and continued with the exercises. At 6 weeks the patient was discharged with all tests normal. He had experienced no pain in either the knee or the back since day 6 from the onset of treatment.

The patient was seen 7 months later with an elbow injury and reported no symptoms in the knee or back since his release.

CASE 3

A 17-year-old girl presented with the primary complaint of pain in the knee with activity and on squatting. History revealed that, while performing as a cheerleader at age 14, she landed on the left knee with the knee in extreme flexion; she had been holding the heel of her left foot to her buttocks with her hand at the time. Arthroscopy had been performed to clean out the debris.

Examination

Pain was elicited on testing of the QF. With manual support of the VMO, pain was reduced by 50%, and performance improved. There was weakness of the popliteus muscle with slight pain on testing. Moderate pain was elicited with pressure on the patella with the knee extended. There was extreme pain with the knee flexed to 100° and lateral pressure on the patella. Palpation elicited pain at the distal right femoral condyle.

Diagnosis

The diagnosis was chondromalacia, unresolved trauma to the right femoral condyle and fasciae due to chronic dysfunction, and unresolved strain of the VMO and popliteus.

Treatment

The knee, lower back, and pelvis were adjusted, and tape support for the VMO and popliteus was provided. Ultrasound was applied over the right femoral condyle, and exercises were prescribed for the VMO and popliteus.

Progress

The tape was removed on day 7. Pain had resolved, and muscles tested at approximately 80% of normal. The patient was released from treatment on day 21 free of symptoms and with all muscles functioning normally.

CASE 4

A 47-year-old woman presented with the primary complaint of pain in the left knee upon squatting and climbing stairs. Secondary complaint (related only on questioning during examination in the erect posture) were severe migrainelike headaches six to eight times per year and less severe headaches more often. She reported random lower back, midback, and cervical pains that came and went no matter what type of treatment was undertaken.

History revealed that the patient had experienced a minor left knee injury 14 months earlier. She had been placed on an exercise program to include the VMO and popliteus muscles.

Examination

On examination, an anatomic short right tibia (1.27 cm) was found. There were no positive findings in the left knee. The left knee also tested stronger than the asymptomatic right knee.

Diagnosis

Dysfunction of the entire body was diagnosed due to the anatomic short leg. Stress to the left knee and compensatory alterations throughout the spine and pelvis were producing the patient's symptoms.

Treatment

After careful evaluation, the patient was fitted with a 0.63-cm heel lift for the right shoe. Exercises for the right quadratus lumborum muscle were also prescribed.

Progress

After 2 weeks, mild exercises for the left quadratus lumborum muscle were added. The knee pain disappeared on day 2 and did not return. Eighteen months after the initiation of treatment, the knee remained pain free. No migraine type headaches occurred, and there were no complaints of pain other than minor compensatory aches, which resolved quickly. There were no severe pains of the spine or pelvis. During those 18 months, the patient was treated 14 times.

CASE 5

A 54-year-old man presented with the primary complaint of pain on the lateral side of the knee on climbing stairs. He gave no other significant history.

Examination

All tests of the knee joint were normal. Testing of the muscles from the foot revealed a weak anterior tibialis muscle. Palpation revealed a hypertonic peroneus longus muscle.

Further testing showed bilateral weakness of the gluteus maximus.

During the examination, the patient was asked whether he had ever had prostate or urethral problems (these would relate to the weak gluteus maximus and anterior tibialis muscles). He admitted to a recent biopsy of the prostate (nonmalignant) and to urinating an average of 42 times per day.

Diagnosis

The lateral left knee pain was produced by a hypertonic peroneus muscle as a result of its reaction to an opposing anterior tibialis muscle weakness.

Treatment

The peroneus longus muscle was stretched, and adjustments were made of all fixations of the foot, ankle, pelvis, and spine. Bennett's neurovascular dynamics reflexes (see Appendix A) over the prostate were performed to reduce edema. At the end of the treatment, the anterior tibialis and gluteus maximus muscles responded at nearly normal levels. The patient could step up as high as the table without pain in the lateral knee. He was instructed in how to apply external pressure to relieve prostatic congestion.

Progress

The patient was a visitor from another state and was instructed to seek a chiropractor in his home state for further treatment. In correspondence 2 months after the one treatment, the patient reported that he had experienced no further knee pain. He was also continuing application of external pressure, and urination was down to 10 to 12 times per day. He had not, however, sought another chiropractor to continue treatment.

Organic Problems and the Knee

Organic problems may produce many signs and symptoms, which may include interference with the normal function of specific muscles. Muscle weakness in the knee area should warn the examiner of at least the possibility of an organic problem. Questioning the patient about other signs and symptoms either will make it mandatory to investigate further or will eliminate organic problems as a cause or as a contributor to the knee problem.

Organ–muscle relationships are controversial. Therefore, before discussing the specific organ–muscle relationships of the knee, it is necessary to relate the author's opinion of the history and theory as well as of methods used to prove or disprove them clinically.

The earliest recorded signs of organ–muscle relationships appeared in drawings of Indian therapeutic yoga exercises. The positions used in therapeutic yoga applied pressure to or stretched specific muscles for each organic problem. The organ–muscle relationships introduced by George Goodheart in the 1960s show a striking similarity to those found in Yogic philosophy.[1,2]

With the introduction of muscle testing, goading of muscle origin and insertion, and organ–muscle relationships, the author, using two other theories, set out to prove or disprove the organ–muscle theory clinically. To my knowledge, no studies have been done to prove or disprove the organ–muscle theory, the fixation–organ theory, or Bennett's neurovascular dynamics (NVD) theories.

An explanation of the author's interpretation of each of the theories is necessary for the reader to follow the methods used.

FIXATION–ORGAN THEORY

For many years, organic "places" have been taught as areas of fixation found by doctors of chiropractic to accompany organic problems. Success in treatment of organic problems has been reported by various clinicians by adjusting the areas indicated. Palmer reported that by adjusting he had restored the hearing of a deaf person.[3] Thus the relationship of an organ to a place started from the beginning of chiropractic in 1895.

Many technique proponents have related various areas of the spine as organic places. These include Biron et al,[1] who referred to the centers and organic places in use by many chiropractors of the time. The most prominent chiropractic system to propose organic places is the Meric system.

The fixation level for an organ may vary from report to report, but they are usually no more than one vertebra apart. Variations of patient anatomy and methods of palpation may account for the differences.

The following are the levels of fixation and the organs related to them as used by this author:

- T1–2, heart
- T3, lung
- T4–5, gallbladder
- T6–8, liver
- T7–8, pancreas
- T7–11, small intestine
- T9, adrenals
- T9–11, kidney
- T12–L1, iliocecal valve and appendix
- L-5, uterus or prostate

Even though there are areas of overlap in the list above, persistent fixation in the area should alert the practitioner to investigate the possibility of organic problems associated with the area. Further investigation may be necessary to prove that the fixation is from organic causes and not a structural fault missed during the examination.

All methods of palpation are fraught with the variables of patient reaction and the examiner's experience and ability. The author prefers palpation of the thoracic and lumbar spine in the supine, non–weight-bearing position for greater accuracy. The distortions and stresses of the prone position for static palpation and the weight-bearing problems in motion palpation interfere with accuracy (see Appendix B for a comparison).

NEUROVASCULAR DYNAMICS

Terrence Bennett, DC, established reflex areas that he felt related to each organ of the body and claimed success in some organic problems by using the reflexes as treatment points.[4]

On the front (Figure A–1) the reflex points are either over the location of the organ or over what Bennett claimed was a reflex from the organ (or valve). The reflex points on the back (Figure A–2) are felt as a tight muscle and are usually sensitive to the patient when palpated. Some of the posterior points coincide with the fixation places. If nothing else had ever come from Bennett's work, the location of the reflex points alone is helpful in diagnosing possible organic problems.

Treatment consists of passive contacts of the two reflexes. With the patient supine, use the right hand and palpate the abdominal area corresponding to the organ that is associated with the area of persistent fixation. With the left hand, contact the area related to the organ along the transverse processes and simply hold. In the author's opinion, this technique helps greatly in decongesting the organ or relaxing the sphincter. The author has helped many patients with known organic problems with the use of NVD as an *adjunct* to adjustive procedures. All reflex techniques should be used only after an adjustment when possible.

Along with the organic place, NVD should be taught as an integral part of diagnosis.

ORGAN–MUSCLE RELATIONSHIPS

Chapman, an osteopath, found that patients with organic problems usually had related sensitive areas, one next to the spine and one on the anterior part of the body (generally different from the NVD areas).[5] Chapman claimed success in treating organic problems by stimulation of the reflexes by goading.

Goodheart introduced to the profession the importance of muscle balance and function as a part of diagnosis and treatment. He found that patients with known organic problems also had specific muscles that tested weak. He also found that stimulation of the reflex areas located by Chapman for the same organ many times resulted in an increase in muscle strength, hence the organ–muscle relationship.

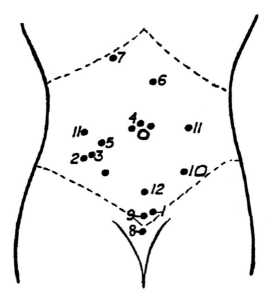

Figure A–1 Anterior reflexes. 1, internal rectal sphincter; 2, iliocecal valve; 3, appendix; 4, small intestine; 5, pyloric valve; 6, pancreas head; 7, gallbladder; 8, urethra; 9, bladder/prostate; 10, ovaries; 11, kidney; 12, uterus.

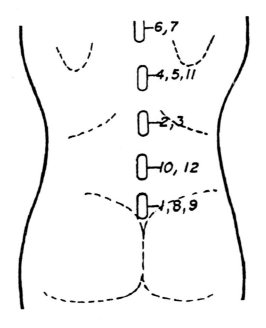

Figure A–2 Posterior contact areas. 1, internal rectal sphincter; 2, iliocecal valve; 3, appendix; 4, small intestine; 5, pyloric valve; 6, pancreas head; 7, gallbladder; 8, urethra; 9, bladder/prostate; 10, ovaries; 11, kidney; 12, uterus.

With further testing, Goodheart found that in the presence of organic problems the reflexes would be present and the muscle would be inhibited from normal function. If the muscle was injured, however, organic function was not affected. He theorized that the common denominator is that the reflex, when stimulated, improves the lymphatic drainage in both the organ and the muscle, hence the term *neurolymphatic reflexes* used in applied kinesiology.

NOTE: The above is the author's interpretation of the work of Bennett, Chapman, and Goodheart and does not necessarily reflect the theories as originally presented. In the attempt to prove or disprove the theory, the neurolymphatic reflexes were not considered, only the muscle weakness, the fixation, and the NVD reflexes.

METHODOLOGY

To prove or disprove the organ–muscle relationship, it was necessary also to prove or disprove the fixation and NVD theories. Several things had to be considered:

- If a patient with organic symptoms presents with a muscle weakness, will the fixation be present? Will the NVD reflex be present?
- If a fixation is persistent and other postural and functional faults have been corrected, will the muscle related to the organ that is related to the fixation be weak?
- If distortions in the posture can be related to one muscle or muscle group, will investigation find that the fixation is present? With further investigation, will the patient have clinical or subclinical symptoms of organic problems?
- If a muscle is inhibited from functioning because of an organ dysfunction, will the muscle respond if the NVD reflexes are used?
- If a muscle is inhibited from functioning as a result of an organ dysfunction, will the muscle respond by adjusting the fixation?

Several methods were used to find the answers. First, students in several postgraduate classes were instructed to dine on spicy Mexican or Italian food for lunch. Upon their return, all the muscles related to digestion were tested and retested during the 3 hours after the meal.

This was not a scientific study; both the subjects and the examiner were aware of the test. Each time this method was used, however, the majority of the muscles that presented weak corresponded with the organ required to function during digestion. As the 3 hours passed, the muscles associated with the stomach returned to normal, and those associated with the pancreas, small intestine, and so forth progressively weakened and then returned to normal. Therefore, it would seem reasonable that, if the muscle is inhibited when the organ is overworked, it should be affected during any dysfunction.

Second, all patients with known diagnosed organic symptoms were checked for fixation, NVD reflexes, and muscle weakness. Fixations were found in the majority of the cases with proven (by ultrasound, radiograph, or computed tomography) organ problems. In several cases where fixations were not present, investigation proved the original diagnosis to be incorrect with the new diagnosis later confirmed by surgery.

The NVD reflexes were present in most proven organic cases. One exception was the presence of stones in the gallbladder. The reflex was not always present without symptoms. A reasonable explanation is that, where stones are present and are not blocking the duct, the reflex would not be triggered. Gallstones are present in many individuals who have never experienced symptoms.

The muscles were affected in almost all the proven organ problems. In the majority of the *proven* organic cases, the fixation, the NVD reflex, and the muscle inhibition were all present.

Third, patients who presented with persistent fixations in an area related to an organ were investigated as thoroughly as possible for other structural faults and, if these were persistent, were investigated for organic problems. The number of clinical and subclinical problems found was great enough to justify the use of persistent fixation as a major sign of organic disease. Some patients without obvious signs and symptoms limited this investigation. The patients could not ethically be referred for investigation without justification. Of course, some persistent fixations could have been, and probably were, compensatory for problems not found in the examination.

One procedure used on several occasions with both students and doctors of chiropractic in workshops is appropriate for this text because it involved the knee. Without explanation, the subjects were instructed to examine each other in the erect posture to identify those with flexion-hyperextension of the knees and then to examine each other in the supine posture with the legs relaxed and suspended by the heels to identify those with flexion-hyperextension without weight bearing. Those with bilateral hyperextension were eliminated from the test. Using only those with unilateral hyperextended knees (27 subjects), the examiners were instructed to test the popliteus muscles bilaterally. Of the hyperextended knees, 96% tested weak compared with the opposite knee (the majority of weak muscles were on the left side). Careful palpation in the supine position found fixations at T4–5 in all cases.

In two groups the author adjusted each patient in the supine position, and in two groups the patients were adjusted by the examiners; both groups had similar results. Upon reexamination, both the weakness and the hyperextension were eliminated in 77% of those adjusted. Of the remainder, six responded when NVD was used. One failed to respond; he reported that he had recently had an injury to the knee.

One can only conclude that, if the gallbladder is under stress, a fixation will be present at T4–5, the popliteus muscle will test weak, the affected knee will be hyperextended, and the NVD reflexes will be present.

By adjusting the T4–5 fixation, a response may be expected by the weak popliteus muscle (there is no direct neurologic explanation) most of the time. Use of the NVD reflex (passive) after all else fails may produce improved function of the popliteus muscle (again, there is no neurologic explanation) and possibly will help gallbladder function.

The value of the above testing is proven often. When an examination reveals a hyperextended knee, a tight, sensitive area is usually present under the right rib cage, and a persistent T4–5 fixation is present. Inquiry into symptoms of gallbladder dysfunction many times surprises patients because they usually do not believe that a relationship exists between the gallbladder symptoms and their structural problems. With the use of organ–muscle relationships and subsequent investigation into the organ problems, the treatment program will be improved.

OPINION

Nothing is absolute. Each reflex, fixation, and muscle test requires judgment on the examiner's part to determine the reflex, the degree of fixation, and/or the loss of normal strength. Accuracy again depends on the experience and ability of the examiner. To cloud the issue further, patient reaction varies from individual to individual.

Most signs and symptoms accepted by the medical community also require this kind of judgment on the part of the examiner. One study in Australia (where there is socialized medicine and one might expect fewer needless surgeries) showed that only 57% of the appendices removed from female patients were pathologic. Other studies in California showed even a lower percentage of accuracy.[6] The accepted signs and symptoms of nausea, elevated temperature, rebound over McBurney's point, and elevated white cell count were the criteria used to determine the necessity for surgery.

If the area of fixation (T-12 and L-19) had been checked, if the NVD points had been palpated and found sensitive, and if the quadratus lumborum muscle had been tested and found

lacking in its normal strength, could needless surgery have been prevented? Would the percentage of pathologic appendices be higher? No one can answer those questions after the fact. If the examiner has the advantage of the additional signs and symptoms provided by the fixation, NVD, and organ–muscle relationships, however, the diagnosis must certainly be more accurate.

There definitely is validity to the existence of an organic place, and it should be taught in palpation and examination and as a part of diagnosis in addition to accepted diagnostic signs and symptoms. NVD reflexes are valuable in the diagnosis and treatment of organic problems and should be taught as a part of diagnosis as well as technique. The organ–muscle relationship is sufficiently correct to include it as one of the signs and symptoms of organic disease and as part of structural analysis.

Using the three theories as a cross-check, I concluded that some of the muscles proposed by applied kinesiologists proved clinically incorrect, although the majority proved correct. Only those proven correct are used in this text (ie, popliteus/gallbladder/T4–5 and quadriceps femoris/small intestine/T7–11). Most of the NVD points coincided with the affected muscles and fixations. The fixations were found to be consistently correct in known, proven organic problems.

None of the above is intended to endorse applied kinesiology or to discredit it. The neurolymphatic reflexes were not used as a part of the tests because my intention was to cross-check NVD. Therefore, the validity of treatment through the use of the neurolymphatic reflexes was not a consideration.

A knowledge of normal muscle function is necessary to enable the examiner to detect malfunction and/or distortion. Determining the cause requires investigation and should include orthopedic testing, neurologic testing, palpation for fixations, muscle testing, and testing of all the reflexes known to be helpful in arriving at a correct diagnosis.

The use of organ–muscle relationships, fixation, and NVD reflexes helps in determining that an organic problem exists, pinpointing the organ involved and adding to existing accepted medical diagnostic signs and symptoms. Their use can only enhance the diagnostic ability of our profession.

REFERENCES

1. Biron WH, Wells BF, Houser RH. *Chiropractic Principles and Technique*. Chicago: National Chiropractic College; 1939.
2. Goodheart G. Applied Kinesiology Notes. Presented at Applied Kinesiology Seminars; 1972–1976.
3. Palmer DD. *The Science, Art and Philosophy of Chiropractic*. Portland, OR: Portland Printing House Co.; 1910.
4. Bennett TJ. *A New Clinical Basis for the Correction of Abnormal Physiology*. Des Moines, IA: Foundation for Chiropractic Education and Research; 1967.
5. Owens C. *An Endocrine Interpretation of Chapman's Reflexes*. Colorado Springs: American Academy of Osteopathy; 1937.
6. Chang A. An analysis of the pathology of 3003 appendices. *Aust NZ J Surg.* 1981; 151(2):169–178.

Several studies have been conducted to determine inter-examiner reliability in palpation. Both static palpation and motion palpation present variables that interfere with reliability.

I used static palpation and, later, motion palpation as taught for many years. I found a more reliable method, however, that I call *passive motion palpation* (for lack of a better term). It is a quicker and far more accurate method of palpation.

Although this text is primarily about the knee, the inclusion of organ problems makes it necessary to refer to palpation of the thoracic and lumbar spine. Before discussing passive motion palpation, a review and critique of static and motion palpation are necessary.

STATIC PALPATION

Static palpation is usually performed in the prone position. This position is convenient because the back may be observed for lesions, muscle bulging, scoliosis, dryness of the skin, and temperature alterations.

The negative aspect of the prone position is that the rib cage is depressed in the front, influencing greatly the rib angle and the transverse process articulation in the thoracic area. The position with the arms suspended forward (toward the floor) stretches the rhomboid and middle trapezius muscles, allowing the scapulae to move laterally and anteriorly around the rib cage. With stretching of the major muscles that secure the scapulae toward the spine, the costovertebral articulation is placed under stress. The stress either causes a reaction of or stretches the levator costarum muscles that secure the rib cage to the transverse processes of the vertebrae. All the above interfere with the accuracy of palpation. The prone position also produces an anterior rotation of the pelvis and an increase in the lordotic curve of the lumbar spine, which interfere with palpation accuracy of the sacroiliac, lumbosacral, lumbar, and lower thoracic articulations.

MOTION PALPATION

One of the great pioneers of our profession, Henri Gillet, DC, developed the type of motion palpation that is currently in use.[1] When performed, it reflects the mobility or lack of mobility of the spinal segments in the sitting position and is an excellent screening technique.

Motion palpation in the sitting position, however, is not without its variables (as shown in several studies), depending upon the body being palpated. In the sitting position the length of the psoas muscles is reduced with flexion of the hip joint. Psoas influence is altered greatly from the erect posture to sitting. If a bilaterally short, hypertonic, or elongated psoas exists, the change would of course be even greater. If an imbalance of the psoas muscles exists, sitting may reveal a normal lumbar spine and no compensatory reaction of the muscles of the lower thoracic spine. On standing, however, the true problem is revealed.

In the presence of a stretched and/or weak quadratus lumborum muscle (invariably found on the side of an anatomic short leg of $1/4$ in or more), the paraspinal muscles are imbalanced. This would also include the iliocostalis lumborum and compensation to allow the erect posture to be maintained.

In the seated position the pelvis is level, but an elongated quadratus muscle may exist on one side. The elongated quadratus lumborum muscle allows elevation of rib 12 on that side and, through the intercostal structures, may allow the entire rib cage on that side to elevate. It also allows the transverse processes of L-1, L-2, L-3, and sometimes L-4 to elevate (some ilia are at the level of the L-4 spinous process and therefore would allow lateral flare of the ilia or shifting to the opposite side of L-4, producing a lumbar scoliosis). With a lumbar scoliosis and an elevated rib cage, many reactions must occur to compensate for the imbalance imposed on the spine.

In the presence of facet syndrome in the lumbar spine with inflammation and edema, weight bearing usually produces reaction and pain. This reaction produces an imbalance in the lumbar spine, again with compensatory reactions throughout the rest of the spine.

Any time weight bearing is involved, any distortion, imbalance, or weakness becomes a major factor in palpation of the structures involved. Palpation by one examiner of structures that are reactive may alter one segment and trigger reactions that of course would alter the findings of a second examiner.

PASSIVE MOTION PALPATION

Passive motion palpation is performed in the supine position. No method of palpation is without its flaws, but palpating the patient in the supine position eliminates the compression of the rib cage, the rotation of the pelvis, the restrictions on the transverse process–rib articulation, and all the weight-bearing problems of the sitting position. It also provides an opportunity to palpate the body in a posture that is as close as possible to the erect posture without weight bearing.

Passive motion palpation is performed with the patient placed in the supine position with the arms across the chest. With the back of the examiner's metacarpals on the table, pressure may be applied to the tissues with finger pressure. This is accomplished by stiffening the fingers, hand, and wrist, using the metacarpophalangeal joints as a fulcrum. With the fingers under the spine, palpation is helped by lowering the examiner's weight and applying pressure through the arms on the spine.

Starting with T-12, bilateral contact on the transverse processes may be made, and anterior glide may be checked. By moving to T-11 with one contact while maintaining contact on the opposite T-12, motion between the two may be checked. The process is then reversed. Oblique mobility may be checked by springing the superior contact superiorly and the inferior contact inferiorly. As palpation progresses up the spine, each segment is palpated. The author uses this method of palpation from the lumbosacral articulation to as high as T-3.

This is not intended to belittle static or motion palpation. Each has its place and time when it is preferred, but for accuracy passive motion palpation is the more reliable method.

REFERENCES

1. Gillet H, Liekens M. *Belgian Chiropractic Research Notes.* Huntington Beach, CA: Motion Palpation Institute; 1984.

Notes

Notes

Notes

Notes